FRONT LINE
Nursing Stories

Making a Difference
An Anthology from the 1940s to the COVID-19 Pandemic

MARIAN FACCIOLO

◆ FriesenPress

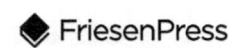

One Printers Way
Altona, MB R0G 0B0
Canada

www.friesenpress.com

Copyright © 2023 by Marian Facciolo
First Edition — 2023

All rights reserved.

No part of this publication may be reproduced in any form, or by any means, electronic or mechanical, including photocopying, recording, or any information browsing, storage, or retrieval system, without permission in writing from FriesenPress.

ISBN
978-1-03-915229-8 (Hardcover)
978-1-03-915228-1 (Paperback)
978-1-03-915230-4 (eBook)

1. Medical, Nursing, Emergency

Distributed to the trade by The Ingram Book Company

FRONT LINE
Nursing Stories

TO: Debbie

Thank you for your valuable contribution to this book

Marian.

Table of Contents

Acknowledgements — vii

Introduction — ix

1. Knowledge for Nurses — 1
2. Why Would Anyone Want to Become a Nurse? — 3
3. Time Travel — 23
4. Relationships — 57
5. Intuition and Experience — 96
6. Abuse and Advocacy — 109
7. Nurses Are People Too — 123
8. Lessons Learned — 142
9. Art Meets Science — 183
10. Challenges to Overcome — 217
11. Ethics in Brief — 223
12. Repairs and Maintenance — 241

Afterword — 268

Acknowledgements

Above all else and most importantly, I would like to thank the many nurses who shared their stories (some shared more than one) for this book. I thank these nurses for their generosity, honesty, and integrity throughout. This book is a collection of nursing stories and, as such, it could not have been written without their contributions. I also want to thank those nurses who shared stories that did not end up being included in the final publication. Each and every story I received encouraged me to keep going.

A special thanks to Maritza McMillen, who was there with me when I initially decided that writing this book was something I was passionate about and wanted to do. Maritza was my Landmark coach. It was during the final workshop that I met her. As the group leader, she provided encouragement and support during the conceptualization and initial plan for my project. Her leadership was both energizing and inspiring.

Jennifer Berry and Colleen Turner were both nurse leaders in the health care system when I initially started this project. Both ladies met me with an open mind and heart. They welcomed me into their agency to talk about my book and ask nurses to share stories with me. Through their efforts, I was able to reach out to some nurses who worked in the community. I thank them for their assistance and their trust.

My sincere thanks to Cyndia Cole, who did a thorough reading of a draft of my book and provided invaluable input. She also linked me with other professionals who contributed along the way. She put me in touch with Piotr Majkowski, who, at the time, was a nurse instructor. He too read through the manuscript, offering valuable feedback. Cyndia also linked me with Jill Mandrake and through Jill to Audrey McClellan. At times, Audrey acted as a sounding board. She helped with editing, and she assisted me to make the book readable for the general public. I would also like to mention my friend Andrea Robarts, who, at times, provided an avenue for me to vent about the process and outcome. She also took some time to review an early draft.

A great big thank you to my friend and painting/drawing buddy Lorraine Maher, who encouraged me to keep plugging away. She was also very effective in convincing a few nurses to share their stories.

I would be remiss if I did not thank my husband Vito, who had to put up with me throughout the entire lengthy process from beginning to publication. He has been my greatest critic and my greatest supporter. I also would like to thank my three sons, Michael, Joseph, and Andrew, for just being there. This book was a labour of love and I tried to keep balanced and enjoy the process. This was not easy, and there were times when this was not the overriding feeling. I feel sure my stress and anxiety surfaced, if only through general osmosis. I thank my family for being there for me and cutting me some slack when I needed it most.

My journey in health care has not been solo. I have worked along side many dedicated service providers who worked tirelessly with their patients and their families.

My deepest gratitude goes out to the many patients and their families whose lives I have had the privilege of being a part of and travelling with along the way.

Introduction

I always had a passion for nursing. When I first thought about putting together this book, I had taken a series of personal growth workshops. During these sessions, I came to the realization that my nursing experiences, and the experiences of other nurses, might be of interest to others. I was on a one-year, self-funded leave from my employment. Although my initial intention was to take a break, smell the roses, travel, and just relax, it occurred to me that it could be the ideal opportunity to write my book. My goal was to finish a first draft by the end of my leave. Of course, this turned out to be far from realistic.

I kickstarted my leave with a wine and cheese party at my home to celebrate my upcoming year off. My work friends were invited. The party also turned out to be a great opportunity to start collecting nursing stories.

Until that time, my nursing career had been long and varied. Initially, I worked on a private medical/surgical unit with people of all ages and conditions. I spent a year of that time in charge on the evening shift. From there, I worked in the labour and delivery room of a large metropolitan city hospital. It was a very busy unit, with women of many different cultures coming to deliver their babies. We had both family physicians and obstetricians do deliveries. In the labour and delivery room, I also worked with a couple of midwives from England. One of my fears was that one day, I might have to deliver a baby. What if the physician did not arrive in time? What if the patient came to our unit crowning and ready to deliver? What would happen if I was the only one available to deliver the baby? One of the midwives sensed my anxiety and understood it, because she had experienced the same fear herself in her younger years. When the opportunity arose, she taught me by standing by me, looking over my shoulder. She coached me. I safely delivered my first baby.

From there, I worked in a hemodialysis unit. The patients there were chronic. During dialysis, the treatment was acute, so the nurses needed to be vigilant for signs of impending shock or side effects of the treatment. The nurses felt valued by the physicians, head nurse, and patients. The chief found ways to show his respect and appreciation for the work we did. We were a close-knit group of professionals. We also became close to our patients, who came in regularly for their dialysis. In some ways, I felt that we were like one big family.

My early years of nursing were in Quebec, but because of the political unrest around the separatist movement for Quebec independence, my husband and I packed up our two boys and moved out west. In Alberta, I found myself working in labour and delivery again, and also teaching pre-natal classes to expectant parents at the local college. After two years, we moved to Ontario, where I continued to work in labour and delivery and post-partum. During my time in Alberta, I became keenly interested in neonatal intensive care. This prompted me to complete a post-grad course in Toronto. A couple of us were offered jobs at the Hospital for Sick Children, where we had done our practicums. I would have loved to work there, but I decided that twelve-hour shifts and a ninety-minute commute each way, with two small children at home, meant it was a sacrifice I just could not make.

I then started working in the community, first as a district nurse and then as a community case manager. As a community nurse, I had the opportunity to work with patients of all ages and at all stages of life. Working closely with families was awesome. Some patients were acute; others chronic and others required palliative care. While there, I worked in many different areas of community nursing, including some time as an educator and as a manager.

I had the opportunity to teach in a nursing program. This change allowed me to learn more about myself, nursing students, and what it's like to function in a teaching and learning environment. I was amazed at the interest level and impact of nursing stories on the students. I also did some curriculum development. This was a place where old and current ideas could be intellectually "trashed" and new, bold ideas proposed. I found it refreshing and rejuvenating. This experience provided me with a much-needed, new and expanded perspective from which to look at the environment and culture of nursing and compare it to where I had come from. This experience made me realize that I missed the closer, direct contact with patients. Subsequently, when I returned to my job in the community, I felt recharged.

In the pages of this book are some of my own stories and many submitted to me by other nurses. The contributors are all Canadian. Many have studied and practiced in different provinces and in different hospitals and community settings across Canada. Although the experiences recounted are varied, they give only a glimpse of the range of nursing duties, at the same time shedding light on what motivates nurses to continue doing what they do in environments that can be challenging and that may not always be supportive. The stories also provide some insight into the lives of nurses as they evolve.

Names and identifying information of the patients and their family have been changed to protect their privacy. Names and descriptions of professionals and others have also been changed to ensure privacy. Only the first names (except for Christine Spears and Stephanie Uhrig) of the nurses telling the stories has been given. A few of the first names have been changed at a nurse's request. There are times when different nurses with the same first name have shared their stories. In such cases, the first name is followed by an assigned initial. The stories and situations are based on real events. In a few stories, the characters and descriptors are a composite of two or more patients, families, and circumstances.

My own voice appears in the book in two ways. I am the narrator of the book. I also tell some of my own stories and disclose personal history so the reader can come to know a bit about my past and how it impacted my nursing career.

Content warning: Some of the stories in this book may cause upset or stress for readers. Please take care of yourself as you read and take a break from reading if necessary. If you need support, please contact your local crisis centre or call a crisis line.

1. Knowledge for Nurses

Generally, the stories shared by nurses in this book do not focus on the science or technical skills required to be an effective nurse. When they are taking courses in a nursing program, student nurses are evaluated academically and are also evaluated for competency with technical skills. Theory and practice are central components that students must integrate in order to graduate. Dr Barbara Carper identifies four knowledge bases for nursing: the science of nursing, the art of nursing, moral or ethical knowledge, and knowledge of the self in relation to others.[1]

The nurse interacts with a patient in order to know and understand them as a person, using the knowledge bases for nursing. A patient interacts with the world or environment as a whole person, with body, mind, and spirit, not just with the medical component that has brought the person into the health care system. Each person is unique and has his or her own values, beliefs, and priorities. Each person makes his or her own choices and decisions. Each person defines health in his or her own personal way because each person's values and beliefs differ.

In my view, for nursing to be therapeutic, it is important that nurses know themselves and their own personal biases. These personal biases can easily get in the way of nursing care.

Throughout the book, nurses speak about their "training" and "education." To give a general overview of how nurses were trained to become certified as

---

[1] Barbara A. Carper, RN, EdD, "Fundamental Patterns of Knowing in Nursing," *Advances in Nursing Science 1* (1): 13–24; reprinted in Janet W. Kenny, ed., *Philosophical and Theoretical Perspectives for Advanced Nursing Practice*, 3rd ed., 3, 22–29 (Toronto: Jones & Bartlett, 2002).

registered nurses, I will share some of my own experiences with the formal education related to nursing in Canada.

When I first entered nursing in the 1970s, a person could become a registered nurse by going through either the diploma program or the degree program. At that time, most RNs went through the diploma programs, which were administered by hospitals.

I originally graduated from the three-year diploma program in Quebec in 1972. This was an apprentice-like program, where nurses studied and lived in residence at a hospital. Student nurses often worked through the summer, with minimal time off. They got practical experience with oversight from their teachers and the staff on the different units. They were not paid for their work, as it was considered part of their studies.

My class was the last one to graduate from our hospital in Quebec. The model was changing and, over time, the hospital-based program was phased out as the nursing program was brought into the college system. Nurses continued to graduate as RNs, but the curriculum was set by the college. Practicums and rotations continued, but not under the direction of hospitals. Nursing students, like other college students, were free to take summer jobs to help support themselves.

Over the past few decades, there has been pressure on diploma nurses to upgrade their education to the degree level. Many believe that the depth and breadth of knowledge and critical thinking skills are enhanced by having a degree. The pressure to move to the nursing degree as the minimal requirement for entry to practice was generally met with resistance by nurses who held only the RN designation. The push to a higher level of education resulted in many diploma nurses feeling devalued, especially those whose life and family situation made it difficult to engage in further education. Many diploma nurses felt anxious about this development, fearing they would either lose their jobs or face limited job opportunities, relegated to less meaningful work or roles. Though most agencies grandfathered in diploma nurses, the anxieties and uncertainties were not easily shed. Of course, the efforts to upgrade did not result in higher income or other compensation, even though they required significant sacrifice in the form of an investment of personal and family time, money, and effort.

2. Why Would Anyone Want to Become a Nurse?

I never intended to become a nurse. I was always going to be a teacher. I'm not sure why, but that is just the way it was when I was growing up in the late 1960s and early 70s. If you were a woman during that time and in the academic stream at school, you either went into teaching, nursing, or studied to become a secretary. Career choices appeared limited for most females.

As a child, I loved painting and drawing, and at one time I thought that it would be fun to be an artist. But how could I make a living doing this? I was reminded that there were a lot of starving artists around. I thought I could perhaps make a living as a graphic artist. But would I be able to pay my rent and other bills? I concluded that this was too risky. I mused about going to teachers' college. One day, my cousin came to visit our family and announced that she was going into nursing school. It was a three-year program and she would graduate as a registered nurse. For a time after her visit, I contemplated this option. I woke up one morning and said, "I think I would like to be a nurse." It was as simple as that.

Several of the nurses I spoke to described what drove their career choice.

MARIAN FACCIOLO

Making a Difference
Lisa's Story

I love being a nurse!

I've been both a pediatric bedside nurse and charge nurse for the unit for more than thirty years, and I honestly couldn't see myself doing anything else. I've experienced some of my greatest joys and some of my deepest sadness, but through the years, it has always been my hope that I could make a difference in the lives of these young patients and their families that I care for.

Several years ago, I was relieving on another unit in the hospital for my night shift. I was approached by a young nurse from this unit who simply asked me if I remembered her. At first, I didn't recognize her, but when she started telling me her story as a patient on my unit, I suddenly remembered this young teenager who had multiple admissions for an unstable heart rhythm, and I blurted, "You're the girl who was unstable on the Esmolol infusion!" I leaped from my seat and hugged her. She told me that I was the reason she became a nurse. It was an incredible feeling knowing that I had inspired this young woman.

She went on to tell me that she had written an article for *Nurses' Week* and posted her story online at the hospital. After reading her submission, I was brought to tears! Her words confirmed for me that I had achieved what I had always dreamed of doing: I had made a difference.

The following is a copy (reprinted with permission) of the story that she published.

"She was my constant."
– Stephanie Uhrig

My nursing profile is going to sound a bit like a missed connection, but I have been wanting to thank this person for years. So this is me working up the courage to do so.

When people ask why I went into nursing, I have to go back about ten years to truly tell the story. At the age of fourteen, I became a patient at SickKids, and that is when I met Lisa, a nurse from 4D. Throughout my various admissions, Lisa was a constant. She would always make time to say hello and come in for a chat. But there was one moment with Lisa I saw how nursing can be a truly extraordinary profession, when an individual can show compassion, strength, kindness, and security even in the scariest of moments. I had just been rushed via ambulance to SickKids and directly to 4D, where several cardiologists and critical care staff were working diligently to stabilize me in one of the worst states I had ever been in, which ended up with a trip to the pediatric ICU. My mother was crying and I was scared but trying to hold it together for her, to show her I was going to be okay. Then in walks Lisa, and I immediately was calmed by the familiarity of her presence. Somehow, in one of my most terrifying moments, she was a beacon of strength and light. She came right to the head of the bed and started talking to me about something as simple as school. While all around me it felt like chaos, she was my constant.

Looking back, I fell in love with nursing when I saw how it could impact another's life. Lisa may not remember me, but I will forever remember her. Because even though it was the simplest of gestures, which I'm sure she does several times throughout a shift, it mattered.

So when I graduated from my BScN, I knew there was only one place I wanted to work. In my years working at SickKids, I have attempted to emulate what Lisa embodied. I show my patients compassion, optimism, laughter and calmness.

I recently had a past patient return, and even though she wasn't my patient, I went in to say hello. She went on to tell me how I had impacted her life, that she tells everyone about me when she talks about her SickKids experience and was so thankful for everything I had done for her. Looking back, I didn't treat her any differently than my other patients. I simply did as Lisa did; I talked with her, showed kindness, and made her feel comfortable in a scary situation.

So Lisa, I am not sure if you will read this, but I want to thank you for inspiring me to become a nurse, showing me what it means to display compassion, kindness, and selflessness. You truly personify what nursing means. I can only hope to keep the cycle of inspiration going into the future.

Reflections
Snowflake's Story

Snowflake (an alias chosen by the nurse who gave me this contribution) shares some of her thoughts about her decision to go into nursing. She was a student in the mid-1960s. Although she acknowledges that it was a difficult time, her story gives us some insight into her choice.

In John Mortimer's book *Paradise Postponed*, the character Dr. Salter states, "Patients and nurses—that's how you can divide the world."

It is much more pleasurable to be a nurse, as opposed to a patient, and some of us simply want to look after others, but it is not an easy ride.

At the age of seventeen, when I chose this path, it seemed the best occupation for me. I couldn't visualize myself as a teacher or an airline hostess or as a secretary. The majority of my high school friends decided to become nurses, although two made the better choice of going to university.

As student nurses, we were told how to do most things, and told frequently, so you didn't have to worry yourself about right or wrong. However, no matter how hard you might try to copy these techniques, there seemed to be lots of room for criticism from your teachers.

I remember one day in the first few months of training when we had a bed-making exam, and I was observed doing so, with our nursing arts teacher checking my every move. She was a much older, cross woman, who took great joy in removing any pleasure from her young students.

In those days, we were required to wear a hairnet. Now, there were two different styles of hairnets. One was the kind that scrunched your hair up into a tight, flat little clump on top of your head, and it came in black or brown. The second type came in a yellowish-blonde colour and was loose, so it hung down on your neck. Neither of these was comfortable. For that reason, I was loath to wear a hairnet, and I remember removing it after the test and putting it in my pocket.

Of course, this did not escape the attention of my eagle-eyed nursing arts teacher, who commanded that I follow her to her office. There she told me to look at myself in her full-length mirror. She said, "Do you think you are playing a fair game?" and "Does that person look like a nurse?" I don't remember what I said, although I have a vague memory of looking at myself through a veil of tears. Later I realized that on that day, and on other occasions when she bullied me, she was cruel and that I hated her.

I stayed in training and eventually the three years came to an end. However, when we have reunions and someone says, "Remember good old ——," I always think about the first-class poop that she was, and how what she taught, she taught with anger, never with a desire to instill a love of nursing in her pupils.

Should I have been a nurse? Probably not, but it did give me a chance to meet many wonderful, caring, and understanding people. So I am grateful. Maybe good old What's-her-name didn't get the opportunity.

MARIAN FACCIOLO

I Want to Make Changes
Kerry's Story

"Hardships often prepare people for an extraordinary destiny."
— C. S. Lewis

I went into nursing after high school because I could get through the program in two years. I was looking for something to get through quickly so I could start working. My parents were telling me I had to go on and do a higher education. This was before the nursing program was in the college or university. It was a diploma program. I went off to the Hospital for Sick Children in Toronto to do my studies.

It was about six months from graduation, and I wasn't doing well at all. I had never been away from home before or even been to a big city. I was a country bumpkin. My good friend from high school also went into nursing at the same time. We had a great time. However, my friend was smart and could go out and party and still maintain good grades. Unfortunately, I was not one of those people. I had to work hard for my grades. It was getting close to graduation, and I knew I needed to pull up my socks and work hard. One of my teachers pointed out to me the differences between myself and my friend. That helped me come to the realization of what I had to do in order not to flunk out and disappoint my parents.

Lenny was my one and only true sweetheart throughout high school. That Christmas, Lenny and I decided we were going to Florida for the holidays. We were going to go in a small plane. He knew an American guy named Kevin who was a rich kid and a pilot. Lenny suggested we get this pilot friend of his and share the cost of gas and go island hopping, visit the Florida Keys. We would have a fabulous time.

The day we left, my parents were excited for us. We all went to Lenny's parents' place for breakfast. Everyone was excited for us. We met the third person, Tony, who was also going to come with us. We didn't really know either Tony or Kevin well. All I knew was they were both good-looking guys. When you are that age, often that is what you are looking at.

It was December 28, and it wasn't a very nice day—it was snowing at the airport. We went to the restaurant to get something to eat, while Kevin went over the flight plan. Tony was with us at the restaurant. He informed us that Kevin was known for doing tricks in the air and diving at his passengers' houses. He said, "I told Kevin, no funny stuff this trip." I agreed with Tony that I didn't want any "funny stuff." Lenny tried to reassure us.

The pilot did not weigh us. He didn't weigh our luggage. It was our first time up in a small plane. Lenny and I really didn't know what to expect. The airport had advised the pilot not to take off, as the weather was getting worse. We did not learn this until later. It was a single-engine plane. Off we went on our adventure.

We were in the airplane for about ten minutes and Kevin was climbing into the air, trying to break through the ceiling of clouds. Tony was in the front with Kevin. Lenny and I were in the back. As he was climbing up, we could hear him trying to get through to the airport. He was asking what the ceiling was at—we could hear all this from the back seat.

Suddenly, out of nowhere, the plane dove and started to spiral out of control. Tony started shouting, "I told you, Kevin—no funny stuff! I told you no funny stuff." But Kevin wasn't saying a word. Then he was touching the dials, moving about frantically, screaming, "Mayday, Mayday!"

Lenny and I looked at each other in astonishment. We looked out the window to see if there was any place we could land. Meanwhile, Kevin continued to call "Mayday!" as the plane levelled out. He said he thought the wings had iced up and he was looking for a place to land or asking to return to the airport. They told him, "No, you can't land here. You have to go to the Buffalo airport."

We could see the thoroughfare way down below. Kevin said we couldn't land there—too many cars—it would be a disaster.

The plane started to spiral out of control again. Kevin yelled at us: "Put your head between your knees, make sure your seat belt is done up, and brace yourselves." Lenny and I just looked at each other. He said to me, "Don't worry, Kerry. You will be able to tell your grandchildren about this."

There was only silence after that. I kept thinking, "Oh God, don't let it hurt... Please don't let it hurt... Please don't let it hurt." I was like a broken record. I'm not sure if the voice was inside my head or if I was saying it out loud. I kept thinking, "This is it. We are gone, we are going to die... we are... finished!"

Total silence.

Finally we were close to the ground. I was watching. At the last minute, I put my head down, bracing for impact. We hit and all I could hear was the sound of crashing, windows popping, metal buckling, seats breaking loose. This was happening in slow motion. Suddenly there was a stillness. It was so quiet, so still, so... eerie. It was now dusk.

I was shocked I was alive. After a few minutes, I thought I heard Lenny trying to say something to me. I woke up—my boyfriend's body and his seat were on top of me. The pilot's body and seat had come back toward me at another angle. I was able to move enough to look outside to see it was dark. We were in some kind of a field with no one around. I kept telling Lenny, "It's okay... conserve your energy... I can't believe we are alive." I kept saying that over and over.

There was no response from Lenny, no response from Tony, and no response from Kevin.

All of a sudden the co-pilot, Tony, started to come to. I looked and noticed that his head looked to be three sizes bigger than it was before. He turned around as he was trying to push the door to get out. That was when I noticed that his eyeball was hanging out. I started to panic as he tried repeatedly to open the door. He was unable to open the door—everything was caved in on us. I was afraid that the plane would blow up.

Out of the darkness, a lady appeared at the broken window. She was peering into what used to be the windshield. She was screaming, "Oh my God... Oh my God!" She was covering her face and screaming. She started to run away.

I cried back at her, "Don't leave us... Please, don't leave us!" I thought maybe she didn't see us or thought we were all dead. I couldn't be sure. What she was doing was running away to get some help. Her husband was with the volunteer fire department, and she was running back to her house to get him. She was running to report the plane crash.

Later, she told us that from the house, she could see a red taillight flickering in the field. She was curious and came to find out what was happening. The plane had landed in their field. Once her husband was alerted, the fire department was called. 911 was called. People started to arrive at the scene.

Because of her reaction, I thought this might be worse than I had originally thought. I didn't realize that my boyfriend was dead. I thought I had heard him trying to talk to me. In retrospect, what I heard was the "death rattle." I heard him take his last breath, but at the time I didn't realize that was what it was.

When the fire department got there, they cut the plane and got Tony out. Then they took Lenny out. Once they took Lenny out, they were able to free me. I could only see that they had him, holding him under his arms, and his head was forward and his legs looked like mine did. I thought to myself, *We can live with broken legs.* At the time, I didn't know he had passed away—I didn't know he was gone.

Then they tried to get me out. I looked down at my leg and saw that my left foot was folded up against my knee. My right leg was broken such that the bone was sticking out and my leg was turned around backward. When they were trying to get me out of the plane, there was a hump under me. They were pulling and catching my leg against it. I kept telling them, "My leg... my leg." The guy finally said, "I see," and someone got over on the other side.

Finally I was out and they were putting me in an ambulance. I was in there, but they didn't have Lenny there with me. I kept shouting, "You can't leave him there!" I could see Lenny in the field, and I kept saying, "You can't leave him there." He was on the field. They told me not to worry, "He is coming... he is coming right behind you." They told me they would be bringing him soon.

They had Kevin in the ambulance with me. I could hear the ambulance driver calling on the phone saying, "Get an orthopedic surgeon ready... ready for a double amputation." I knew they were talking about me. I saw my legs. I was upset but kept thinking, "I am going to lose my legs, but I am alive."

We got to the hospital and the last thing I remember is the doctor looking at me. The nurse was asking me about my religion. The doctor, without any medication, grabbed my foot and pulled it down—whoop... one huge whoop and pulled it down. He did this quickly and without any hesitation. All I could see was a clock over my head that read six o'clock. I thought I had passed out.

They told me I had not passed out, but apparently, I had some real choice words for that surgeon. They informed me I was cursing and swearing!

I was brought to the operating room and given a spinal anesthetic. They did not have a choice. They knew that I had recently eaten a big steak dinner. With a general anesthetic, a patient must not have anything to eat or drink for a specified time before the surgery. They were concerned I might aspirate. They were also worried about possible internal injuries.

I don't remember my parents arriving, but I was in a hospital in the States. I remember waking up and not feeling anything from the waist down. I was being moved from one place to another on a stretcher. My mother was walking beside me. I told her, "They took them both, mom… they took them both. They took both my legs."

She said, "Honey… no, they didn't. Look down, you have two casts on." She told me the doctor had said that it was a good thing I had not been into drugs or anything, because that meant the antibiotics they gave me were very effective. He said they were concerned they would have to amputate. My legs had gone through the bottom of the plane, and they were sitting in mud. My system was open and exposed to toxins while my leg was ripped apart. They were worried about the toxins going into my bloodstream.

I kept asking about Lenny. My mother kept saying, "Kerry… he's okay."

Later, I saw something on the news. I could have sworn it said, "One dead, three critical!" Right away the nurse came in and said, "Turn that off." I wasn't really listening until she said, "Turn that off." The nurse turned it off. I asked the doctor about Lenny the next day. There was still no explanation. They did something strange. They brought a nurse from another unit who I had never met and would never see again. One morning, I woke up and the nurse was sitting beside my bed. I said, "Hello," and she introduced herself as a nurse from another unit. She asked me how I was doing. Then she told me she needed to tell me something that would be really hard for me.

I didn't graduate that year. I was in the hospital for six months, and in and out of the hospital for a couple of years after that. I had to have bone grafts on both legs, and it took a long time. I had to learn to walk again. The doctor told me I would never go back to nursing. He said it was not a possibility—I would need to have a sedentary job. Well, you never tell Kerry that she can't do something. I have a stubborn streak, and if you tell me I can't do something, I will prove you wrong.

While I was in the hospital, I had a lot of bad experiences. I had a lot of pain. As a nursing student, I knew that they could only give you pain medication every so often. I knew this and would try to hold out for that pain medication as long as I could. In my mind there was no sense asking for it as I couldn't get it, so I would wait. Then I got labelled as a drug user and a clock-watcher. They felt I was waiting for each analgesic to anesthetize myself and not deal with the situation. This wasn't the case—I was in a lot of pain and was trying to be a good student nurse. This happened a lot. There were times when I needed to void, with two legs in casts, and waited for someone to come to assist with a bedpan.

This was when I made up my mind that I was going back to nursing. I was going to be a head nurse and I was going to make sure that every nurse on my unit treated people right. There would be no such thing as "clock-watching for your pain medication." I was determined to do that. The doctor told me I was setting myself up for disappointment. I told him I was determined to try.

I had a brace built for one of my legs. They sent me to the best, Dr. Salter from Sick Kids Hospital, who was world renowned for orthopedics with pediatric patients. By this time, I was twenty years of age. The brace he built for me looked like a prosthesis with a foot and a shoe on it. You slid your leg into this shoe and brace. It took all the weight on my knee, rather than the ankle.

I returned to nursing with a new enthusiasm. I knew what I wanted and was ready to do it. I graduated with fabulous marks—a mature student with almost a lifetime of experiences behind me. I can't imagine doing anything else with my life. Those experiences I had helped me become the person and nurse I am.

I ended up having to start over again, and this time it took four years, because the nursing program had become a university program. I graduated from Toronto General and Ryerson in 1979 and got a position at UCLA medical centre. My brother-in-law ended up working on the bone marrow transplant unit at the same place. This is how I launched my career.

I had lived in a small town, and everyone knew Lenny and me. In some ways, this made it more difficult, as everyone knew what had happened. It was a horrific thing and it took me a long time to get over it. But when I was ready, I needed to move on with life and needed to break from all the reminders.

I did end up returning to Toronto from California and worked at Princess Margaret Hospital as a nurse manager on the leukemia/lymphoma unit. We had a fantastic group of nurses. We had so many wonderful evaluations from patients and families. When I needed to, I told staff my story. I did reach my goals.

I am married now. Lenny's parents were there at my wedding. Lenny's brother became a pilot and was the first person to take me up in a plane after my experience with the crash.

These days, when I am on a plane and someone near me is fearful, I just tell them that I am living proof of someone who survived a plane crash and lived to tell about it. I ask them if they have ever heard of someone being in two plane crashes in their lifetime.

I Knew My Path
Dayle's Story

I was just ten or twelve years old when my grandfather became sick. He had been unwell for a couple of years. They had done a lot of tests. He was short of breath (SOB) and they didn't know why. He was a Christian man—he never did without, but did not live lavishly. My grandmother was a stay-at-home mom. Early in their marriage they did some farming, but later, they ran a Christian resort. I was close to my grandparents. They lived about a two-hour drive from us, and as children, we stayed with them for at least two weeks in the summer and saw them for long weekends. They looked after us when we visited them.

My grandfather was a self-employed contractor and didn't have any benefits when he was diagnosed with scleroderma. He had to sell some of his possessions in order to be able to manage financially.

There was a slow, steady deterioration in his condition. He continued to be SOB and was started on oxygen. He had difficulty swallowing and needed a G-tube [a gravity or gastrostomy tube, which takes food directly into the stomach] inserted. The nurse did home visits and showed my grandmother how to clean and dress the G-tube site, make up the saline solution, and sterilize the wound forceps. One day when I was visiting and she was going to do the procedure, I mentioned to my grandmother that I would like to try it. She demonstrated how to hold the forceps, wring the saline out of the swabs, and go from clean to dirty. She had me wash my hands thoroughly and handed me the forceps. I was shaking. I reached out so gently and quietly. My grandfather barked at me! I was surprised and jumped. He laughed and laughed. "You're not hurting me, Dayle." He was such a kind and gentle soul.

About two years later, he passed away. In the meantime, although sick, he kept busy. He liked to keep busy in his workshop. He loved building things; he would go in there with his oxygen and continue to work. I remember all the good things about him. He kept active, and mentally he was sharp.

I wasn't there when this next thing happened. I am told he had his work gloves on when he was using a saw and ended up amputating four of his fingers on his dominant right hand. He was already compromised, and then this happened. They were only able to reattach his pinky finger. I think his thumb only had minor damage. He ended up having hand splints made, and a special one that he could use to help him write. An occupational therapist was involved with making the splints and teaching him to write, using the palm of his hand to guide him. A visiting nurse was arranged to do the dressing. His hand was a mangled mess. I never did that dressing.

My grandfather was very proud of me and he told me so. Before his death, he spoke with each of his children and grandchildren individually. He then wrote a letter to his family and had one of his daughters read it at his funeral. In this letter, he spoke to each one of us again. In his words to me he mentioned his memory of me doing his dressing when I was young. He mentioned how proud he was of me and his desire for me to be a nurse. At that time, I was already in my first year of nursing.

From my perspective, my grandfather went through a lot. My grandmother was his caregiver. She did it with such grace and, from my child perspective, without caregiver stress. This was my view as a child looking in. I watched my grandfather going through illness and disease and healing and recovery. The things I witnessed I thought were amazing. From the time I was able to do that first dressing until after his passing, I knew that nursing was what I wanted to do with my life. I saw it, was interested in all of it—the physical, emotional. I saw the challenges as the disease progressed. He went in and out of hospital with recurrent pneumonia. I saw how his body changed. Over time, he got increasingly frail, his shoulders and arms got smaller and smaller, his skin colour worsened as his breathing and condition deteriorated. He had a large belly. As a kid, I remember thinking, "As long as he has that big belly..."—he looked good. Now that I am a nurse, I understand the side effects of the steroids he was on. I realize that it was those effects I was watching.

I Watched a Soap Opera
Patricia's Story

Why did I go into nursing? Honestly, the straight answer is because of my beloved grandma. I enjoyed spending a lot of time with her when I was a teenager. We would often watch the TV soap opera *General Hospital*. My grandma had a stroke when she was in her sixties, which left her paralyzed on one side. I would try to help her as much as I could, including by cleaning her home. She had many children and grandchildren, and she had always hoped someone would go into nursing, so I decided that would be me, given how glamorous the profession seemed to be on *General Hospital*.

Off to nursing school I went and quickly realized things were not quite how I had envisioned. I called my grandma and let her know I was having to get up at 5 a.m., and that working in the hospital was not at all like I had seen on TV. However, I did work hard, and reality set in along the way. I was thrilled to have my grandma at my graduation, and she was thrilled to be there.

So began my thirty-year nursing career, of which I am very proud. Proud to have cared for so many people and worked with many dedicated colleagues. Proud to have advocated for so many people and proud to develop so many effective relationships with families, caregivers, and other professionals.

Why did I leave nursing in 2020, at age fifty-four and after thirty years? Honestly, I had given my all to this profession and could no longer continue with the increased demands, which, at times, would jeopardize my ability to provide safe and effective care. Finally, feeling unsupported, I felt I had no choice but to leave while I was still intact. I look forward to my life's Second Act.

What Comes Next?
Sharon M.'s Story

I grew up in the 1950s in a very dysfunctional family. My mother was abused by my father, and I was as well. My family was on welfare for a long time. My mother had a good friend named Mrs. C., who was very supportive of my mother and our family when we went through all those difficult times. I don't know how we could have managed those early years without her and her help. I was able to get through elementary and high school. Sometimes I wondered if I would make it, given all the challenges.

I ended up doing an extra year of high school and then worked as a waitress to earn money for my schooling. I was eighteen months from graduating with a bachelor of education from McGill University. I did some supply teaching of Grade Three in my hometown. It was difficult, because I had babysat most of these kids before this classroom experience. My role with them was different from what they had known before this. My classroom work did not go well. I felt it was an absolute disaster. The kids were out of control. I did not enjoy teaching in any way and could not think of anything positive about the experience. I felt like a failure. I decided not to pursue this career.

There were not a lot of options in the early 1970s. After consideration, I decided to try nursing. I spoke with my mother's friend, Mrs. C. She was a wonderful person. She was also a nurse. Understanding who and what type of person she was inspired me to try nursing. I looked up to her.

I ended up enrolling in the nursing program, thinking I would hate working with kids. I was ready to get my practicum over with and hopefully find my place working with adults. I graduated as a registered nurse, and several years later, completed my bachelor of science in nursing. To my surprise, I chose to work with children for the duration of my long and satisfying career.

Nursing Saved My Life
Susan's Story

This is a story that is very personal to me. It is a story of deep grief and sorrow. I really don't know where to begin. As I think back and reflect on it, I can feel my gut churning and wrenching. I'm not sure anymore what part is personal and what part is professional. I feel like I have been sucker-punched, or maybe that someone has successfully eviscerated me and slowly put me back together. When that happens, a person is never quite the same. It is hard for me to separate the personal and professional, as they weave together like a tightly knit scarf that circles my neck and could, with little provocation, suffocate me.

I absolutely don't know where to begin. Few people are aware of my story. I can say that nursing saved my life.

I first encountered the idea of nursing as an infant when I was receiving care myself at Sick Kids Hospital. I'm sure I carry memories of this time that have been incorporated into my being. I heard from my mom about the experience, so her thoughts and expressions of events probably planted the seeds for what I would eventually choose to do with my life.

When I was twelve years old, my father committed suicide. He was mentally ill for a very long time. He was an aircraft mechanic in the Second World War. He committed suicide the same year that his younger brother committed suicide. As a twelve-year-old, I came home from school and discovered a grisly scene. It was the end of my childhood. Back then, there wasn't a lot of counselling. We just got on with our lives. My one sister was gone from home and the other sister was in university. It was just my mother and me left at home. I did well in high school and finished Grade Thirteen in four years. I then worked for a couple of years. Then, I decided to go into nursing.

During my second year of nursing, there was a patient on the night shift who hung himself. He was a young man who had AIDS. It was in the early days of AIDS, and he was admitted to the hospital with fever not yet diagnosed (NYD). People with this diagnosis were dropping like flies. He hung up his oxygen mask and left a note. I was making my rounds and he wasn't in his bed. He wasn't in the kitchen. He wasn't in the lounge, sitting by the window overlooking the city. I looked around for him. He wasn't anywhere to be found. I searched everywhere for him. I tried to open the door to the bathroom. I was able to pry the door open enough to turn on the light. His body was collapsed against the door, preventing me from opening it. I screamed. I tried to pry the door open and called for help. We coded him, but it wasn't successful. They intubated him but weren't successful in reviving him. While all this was happening, I was seeing my own father, rather than him. I was thinking, "How can lightning strike twice?" But obviously it does.

After that, I worked at various nursing jobs and nursing positions all over the country. When my boys were young, I was working in a hospital in Fredericton. An orderly came into the room where I was working to help me with a patient. He told me that someone had come into the emergency department the night before. He wasn't a patient, but a stranger who had come into the emergency room and shot himself in the washroom. I didn't really think much of it at the time. I went for my break and returned to the unit. When I returned, it was as if I had been frozen in time. There was a social worker on the unit who recognized what was happening with me. I was replaying the scene and it was as if a switch had been turned on, replaying the same event over and over.

In the next few years, I must have encountered five or six people who I knew had lost someone to suicide. There was the twenty-two-year-old son of a friend of mine, the occupational therapist who worked at the hospital, the wife of a neighbour, and others. I was always able to provide comfort and support to them. At the same time, I attended a conference on parish nursing. The woman sitting beside me said that a neighbour of hers—a woman with several children—had been abandoned by her husband. What struck me was the abandonment. Something in her story reminded me of my own situation. We connected and shared our stories. She said that we have to do what Jesus would have done and that, "You are going to let me take you to the priest."

I said there was absolutely no way that was going to happen. But for some reason, I did let her lead me to a meeting with the bishop and Anglican minister, and they prayed. I don't know what happened, but during this encounter, I saw a vision of my dad in the arms of an angel. Surrounding my dad was this beautiful light. It was very comforting for me at the time. It has been comforting since and through all these years.

Now where it has affected me is in the care of the elderly, and particularly, working with veterans and people with mental health issues. I just think that all those experiences from my past haven't been for naught. So I share my story with people and help them come to terms with their own feelings of loss and pain and the effects of war on people. It isn't just the generation of my father, but it is every war and conflict that inflicts that kind of injury on people.

A friend recently asked me how I could have gone through all that and still be able to provide comfort and support to people. I told them I don't usually cry about it, as I am while telling this story now. I do think I have a strong faith. I wish there was a better way. I wish the medications had been better years ago when my dad needed them. I wish people could get the help they need to get their problems sorted out. I agreed with my friend who suggested that my personal experiences helped me connect with people in pain. I believe that when I open up and tell them my own story, they know I understand their pain. There is a trust factor.

The pain is always there for me. I have this necklace that I wear most of the time. When we were children and were travelling somewhere with my dad, he would hum certain tunes and point out the owls, hawks, eagles, and other raptors. He would always spot them. I do that now too. I find myself always trying to spot things. I told my girlfriend about it and she made me this necklace. She carved it from antlers, and there is an imprint of an eagle on it. It provides a comfort to me. It provides me with a feeling of protection. I always try to make sure I wear it when going into a vulnerable situation. I know it sounds superstitious, but it means a lot to me. I believe it embodies my dad and does offer me protection.

After my dad died, if it was not for nursing, I believe I could have been a street kid. I could have gone either way. I went into nursing, and so here I am, telling you my story.

Father Father

I am my father's daughter, the lessons branded within me
Your self-willed death, your bloody hand, the pain crusted within me
Where had you been to wound me so, so cruel to so demean me
Your death before my eyes, your intention to destroy me?
It set my path, the loveless path, no hope of growth within me.

It was the longest journey to heal my soul
To know the truth of death gone awry
That tore my fractured will to thrive.
Release me, Lord. Unburden me this agony.

Your death, your death, restored the life within me
I chose the nursing path to nurture and to save me.
Through others' pain, through others' death, I found the will within me
To heal the sick, to honour you and to love the soul inside me.
I am my father's daughter, your love I carry with me.

– Anonymous

The stories in this chapter speak to the differences that motivate people to pursue the same path. Stephanie was inspired by Lisa. Kerry, on her first attempt with nursing, thought that becoming a nurse would satisfy her parents. Life events changed everything for her. Her resolve and tenaciousness allowed her to become a nurse determined to make a difference. Nursing helped keep Susan from falling apart, while Snowflake was motivated by the need to help others. Sharon first chose teaching, but found it unsatisfying. She found her niche in nursing on her second attempt at a profession. Dayle knew from a very young age that nursing was her calling. Patricia's motivation appears frivolous and shallow, but her decision thrust her into a position to impact many people's lives.

3. Time Travel

"The best way to find yourself is to lose yourself in the service of others."
– Mahatma Gandhi

In this chapter, individual nurses from the 1940s and later share their views and perspectives on nursing as they experienced it during their time. Miae tells the story of Florence Nightingale and what life was portrayed to be like for nurses more than a century ago. Although this is not a comprehensive historical account of nursing, it does provide insight into each nurse's experience and perception of the times.

An Overview
Miae's Story

The following is part of a speech presented by Miae in May 2011 to a group of her colleagues during Nurses' Week celebrations. At the time, Miae was a nurse working as a case manager in a community setting. The local member of the provincial parliament was in attendance, as were many of the nurses who worked for the community organization.

MARIAN FACCIOLO

Florence Nightingale was born May 12, 1820, in Florence, Italy, the city she was named after. Because of her father's futuristic thinking about the education of women, she and her sister were well educated in the different ancient and modern languages, history, and music. They were also well-travelled.

One account of Florence Nightingale's early training as a nurse in Germany's Institute for the Training of Deaconesses is the following:

> The trainees were up at five a.m., ate bread and gruel, and then worked on the hospital wards until noon. Then they had a ten-minute break for broth with vegetables. Three p.m. saw another ten-minute break for tea and bread. They worked until seven p.m., had some broth, then Bible lessons until bed.

Of that experience, Florence wrote, "The world here fills my life with interest and strengthens me in body and mind." She was a dedicated and spiritual woman.

Florence Nightingale developed friendships in high ranks of society, gained prominence through her study of hospital and health matters during her travels to Germany, Ireland, England, France, Italy, and later Egypt.

She is well-known for her work as a charge nurse in the Crimean War in 1854, as well as her involvement with the sick and poor in London's workhouses. Through these experiences, she bore witness to the effects of socio-environmental conditions, such as poverty and lack of sanitation, on health and disease. She provided direct nursing care and simultaneously used her social connections and nursing expertise to write to politicians advocating for changes to improve workhouse conditions and the treatment of the sick and poor. She was emphatic about quality nursing and proper training of nurses and what is now termed "evidence-based practice."

Two hundred and one years after Florence Nightingale's death, we stand here at our community workplace as case managers. Whether we do home visits or speak with our clients and caregivers on the phone, we continue to bear witness to the close association of health, poverty, marginalization, and sickness. We provide case management service, nursing assessment, care that is evidence based, counselling, a listening heart, and help to solve complex problems. We as nurses continue to be a voice that dialogues with the politicians at all levels of government to advocate for health.

As we work Monday to Friday or Sunday to Sunday (depending on the area of work within the organization), it is easy to get lost in the current monotony or mediocrity. I tell the inspirational story of Florence Nightingale during Nurses' Week to help us not forget who we are. We are nurses. Let's not forget the value that the profession and discipline of nursing contributes to the individual, community and global health.

Over time, the goal of nursing has remained constant and consistent with the views of Florence Nightingale. The concept of health has broadened to include a person's body, mind, and spirit. Our core role is to help people recover from illness, injury and promote health and healing. To accomplish the goals of care, the means have undergone dramatic changes both in process and in the tools that are used. I look back over the past thirty years and feel that change has moved, and continues to move, at warp speed.

Nursing in the 1940s
Evelyn's Story

Evelyn was ninety-two years old when she submitted this story. She tells about her life and why she decided to go into nursing. She graduated in 1943 and gives us a glimpse of what it was like living then and her decision to become a nurse. She describes a hospital-based program that she refers to as "training."

My name is Evelyn and I am a graduate of Victoria Hospital in London, Ontario. I was the fourth child in a family of seven children. I had two older brothers, an older sister who died when she was six, and two younger sisters.

MARIAN FACCIOLO

We lived on a farm in rural Ontario. I attended primary and high school located about seven miles from where we lived. My dad died of a ruptured appendix at age thirty-one, when my mother was pregnant with my youngest sister. My mother had only a public-school education, so she had to work at manual jobs, like house cleaning and factory and farm jobs. It was the Depression, and times were hard. With help from families and neighbours, our family survived. Of course, we all worked as soon as we were able. We picked strawberries for two cents a quart basket or worked in tobacco at two dollars a day. Even with this, we struggled. Mom was determined to keep us all together. It was the greatest gift she could give us. The other was that she made sure we always knew we were loved.

She wanted her girls to have an education, because she felt life might have been easier for her if she had more education. So the girls all got through public school. My brothers had only one year of high school and then they dropped out and found jobs.

I loved school and was a good student. I started high school at eleven years and finished at seventeen. We had to be in our nineteenth year to go into nursing training, so I worked for a year in a tobacco factory in the winter and a store in the summer.

My first visit to London was traumatic. The furthest I had ever been from home was to Detroit, which was thirty-five miles from my home. Prior to my admission to nursing, I needed to have a health assessment, which included a physical examination. I was petrified. I was directed where to go to have this done in London. I was greeted by the doctor, a kindly old man who said, "Go behind the screen and take your clothes off." I stood there, with my mouth hanging open I'm sure, and said, "ALL OF THEM?"

Before I was accepted into the nursing program, I had to have my tonsils out. At the time, I was staying with my brother, who was living in town. I walked to the doctor's office, had chloroform, had my tonsils removed, and walked back home. It cost me twenty-five dollars for the surgery. Of course, I didn't realize at the time that I could have bled to death.

I always knew I wanted to be a nurse. In those days, you had three choices: teacher, nurse, or secretary. So in September 1940, the big journey began. I saved money to buy my own books and uniforms. We had a blue-and-white-striped dress with short sleeves and a white apron over that. It measured twelve inches from the floor. Black shoes, long stockings, a white starched collar, and cuffs on the sleeves completed our uniform.

We lived in residence, two people to a room. We worked twelve hours with a two-hour break either in the morning or afternoon. Along with classes and time on the wards, the days flew by. I was so homesick. I think my mother wrote me every week. I wasn't the only one who was homesick.

In training, we had to have rotation on every service: operating room, gynecology, medicine, surgical ward, dietary, etc. We spent about six weeks on every service. My favourite was the new baby nursery. We got five dollars a month and room and board. Our personal hours were very restricted. We had to be in every night at ten p.m. Once a month, we could be out until midnight. Smoking was a no-no! Some of the girls smoked. There was always a window open if someone stayed out late. On the whole, we got along quite well. In retrospect it was like a big family. We shared our clothes, our money, especially if someone had a date. There was a "housemother" who watched over us and had her office at the front entrance. You had to check in and out of residence.

I completed all my book learning in eighteen months. Once courses were completed, students often had "charge duty," especially on wards. The wards were big rooms with several beds, sectioned off by curtains that could be pulled around them. Supper came in a metal wagon (I can't think of the name) with hot water and the food in canisters, kept warm by the hot water. Every night, someone would put the coffee in a big blue pot that sat on the stove all night. I guess it was the smell, but I have never been able to drink coffee since then.

There was an underground tunnel from our living quarters to the hospital, and we went over to where we lived and had our meals in the dining room. What can I say? They were hospital meals and they were "adequate." It was always good to eat somewhere else. After two months, we got our caps, and it was a real big deal. I was assigned to a room with men with broken legs, broken backs, etc., and when I came in with my cap on, they had taken a newspaper and made a dunce cap. I could have killed them.

Three years seemed to be a long time, but it went quite quickly, and I graduated in 1943.

MARIAN FACCIOLO

It was wartime, and we did not have any antibiotics until penicillin came along. We had babies die because of the wrong Rh factor [blood group] and we didn't know why. Finally, the Rh factor was isolated in the blood. At that time, people still died of pneumonia. Patients who had surgery were brought back to the ward, and we took care of them as they recovered from anesthetic. Good nursing care was most important. If you cared for someone who got bedsores, you were in trouble. Men who had prostate surgery and couldn't void would stand up by their beds, and we had to support them. When we had a patient die, two nurses would prepare the person to go to the place where they were kept until they were buried. The first time you had to do this was quite scary.

After my husband went overseas, I worked from the registry as a private nurse in the hospital and in homes. [A registry is a private company that had a roster of nurses who would do shift nursing in different hospitals. Some nurses made themselves available for only one hospital or a couple of hospitals or specified certain shifts or certain areas they were prepared to work in, while other nurses were open to any hospital and any nursing duty at any time. The registry ensured all nurses were in good standing and had proper licensing.] Sometimes you were on a case for weeks doing eight-hour shifts. From what I recall, we made seven dollars a shift.

Wartime was hard. We had some restrictions on certain foods, like sugar and butter. And there was always the fear that your loved one wouldn't come back. Thank God mine did. We were married fifty-four years, and he died fifteen years ago from a massive stroke.

After he came home, I continued to work until we had our family of three boys. I was home for fifteen years with them. When I went back to work, I had to be retrained for ICU, recovery, dialysis, etc. I worked at Victoria Hospital as a relief nurse for several years. Then I got a call from the Red Cross Blood Department and worked there for fourteen years. We collected blood in the southwestern area of Ontario. It was a great way to finish my career.

The nurses who I trained with and graduated with had many reunions. The sixtieth was our last. Living in residence and being in training is like having another family. We lived together for three years. At present, there are still five members of my class living.

I never had any regrets about my career choice. It was hard work and there were good times and bad, but I was always proud to be a nurse. When you live day in and day out with illness and death, you can't help but wonder what it is all about. For me, it was always God's work I was doing. I sometimes saw what I considered miracles. I remember one lady who was dying. Her son came from out of town to visit. An intern got him to sign a request for an autopsy. That lady got better and went home. Another lady had abdominal surgery and they said she was full of cancer. They just closed her up. She went home and lived for seven years. During my nursing career, I witnessed some miracles along the way. These ones I mention I feel were "another miracle."

Nursing in the 1950s
Shirley's Story

Shirley talks about her memories of her nursing education in the 1950s. Like Evelyn, she refers to this as her "training." She mentions all the odd jobs that nurses did in the hospital, which were tacked on to the central nursing role. Hospitals didn't have the auxiliary staff they do today. For example, nurses became porters when this was needed. They delivered and retrieved the meal trays. Shirley says that things started to change for nurses in the 1960s. She remembers that this was when she started to get vacation time.

Nursing back in the 1950s wasn't like it is today. I graduated from the old Grace Hospital in Winnipeg, Manitoba, from a three-year diploma course. It was a general hospital that was accredited. We took our theory and practical at the hospital and wrote our exams at the University of Manitoba.

There were rules for us when we were students, and we needed to comply. For example, we had to be in student residence by ten p.m. every night. We were allowed one overnight away from residence each month. That amounted to twelve overnights a year in total. Because my home wasn't in the city, I rarely saw my family. Each year we were given a couple of weeks' holidays. We often worked both Christmas and New Year's Day. Even in my last year, I did not get Christmas off. Seldom did we luck out and get the statutory holiday off. Our family and boyfriends had to be very understanding.

As students, we started out on probation. Three months after probation, we received our caps if we made it through. At the end of six months, we wrote qualification exams at the university. If you didn't pass these, you were out of training. Two students in our class didn't pass that year and had to come back with the next class being admitted.

Our hospital was staffed on each floor by a registered nurse, and the rest of the staff were students. By the time we had written our qualification exams and were juniors, we were taking on a lot of responsibility. We worked days, evenings and night shifts, and on evenings and night shifts there were no charge nurses [nurses in charge of the specific floor or unit]. There was one supervisor for the entire hospital. You had to call her if you felt someone required a narcotic and for any major problem.

I was a junior when I first had to work the night shift. I had a really hard time sleeping during the day. Students who were working days came over to the residence for lunch and to go to class. It was noisy. Students who were working evenings were up walking around in the dorm, running water, talking and yelling and having fun. They were letting off steam. After about eight days without sleep, my neck became very stiff. I felt quite sick. There was a polio epidemic at the time. They figured I was getting polio when I was so sick. Finally, I was diagnosed as being sleep-deprived. I never did sleep very well when working nights.

In the 1950s, there were no aides to take flowers in and out of patients' rooms, dust furniture, etc. We were expected to do these tasks on top of the nursing care. Our attention to these added tasks was monitored and evaluated along with our ability to do the nursing care for our patients.

One of our classmates dropped out of training when we started practical procedures. She had not realized she would have to carry and clean out a bedpan. She thought she was going to be able to walk around in a crisp clean starched white uniform. This wasn't the case.

FRONT LINE NURSING STORIES

I remember being apprehensive when we were learning to give hypodermic needles. Usually, you practiced the technique by injecting oranges. Our training instructors decided that we would have to give them the injection instead. We used sterile water to inject. I was afraid I would hit a blood vessel. I remember one of my girlfriends said, "Oh, don't be so silly. That won't happen." Guess who hit a blood vessel? And it wasn't me.

We had classes for the practical training, and we had to demonstrate that we could do all procedures proficiently in class. Then our instructors monitored us several times while we did them with our patients. They would sign off on us when they thought we were ready to do them on our own.

Bed baths were a major production. This was one of the first things we learned to do. Our training included the process of doing it and how to do it differently depending on the mobility and function of the person in the bed, but most importantly, how to preserve the dignity and privacy of the person in the bed. There was an art to setting up for a bed bath and for the procedure itself. It all depended on the amount of assistance the patient required. Sometimes, setup was all that was needed. Other times, patients required complete care, including turning, positioning, mouth care, skin care, and peri-care [cleaning the private parts]. Privacy, dignity, and respect were highlighted. Back rubs and personal care were offered in the morning and in the evening. Nurses made the beds, and it was expected they would be wrinkle free. Nurses were expected to wash their hands before and after every procedure. This helped to keep the infections out of the hospitals.

Our operating room and labour and delivery room training was intensive. I believe it was really good. As students we had to "scrub in" for many major and minor operations. We were expected to "scrub in" for many births as well.

The operating rooms were scrubbed down every day with disinfectant. The nurses did it. This included scrubbing the instruments, glass syringes, operating stands, and floor basins. It included most of the equipment. Once scrubbed, the instruments and syringes were sent to be autoclaved [sterilized]. At that time, in the hospital, all dressing trays, catheterization trays, and other equipment were scrubbed and autoclaved. Nurses did all of this. There was no throwaway equipment. Sterile gloves were used for sterile procedures, but not for general nursing. You were expected to wash your hands between all procedures. I don't remember that the infection rate from cross-contamination or hospital-acquired (nosocomial) infections were an issue.

After students spent a short time working in the operating room, there was an initiation process. A few days after your first couple of cleaning sessions, when you least expected it, senior nurses would grab you and tie you to a floor basin. They would put ether over you and put you on an elevator, making sure you stopped at every floor. It was just what they did to you as a novice in the operating room area.

In my estimation, we got very good training in all departments. We did our placements with children and communicable diseases in other hospitals. That was because we did not have these specialty areas in our general hospital. When I was at both hospitals, I worked with polio patients who were in iron lungs. At the children's hospital, I worked with a nine-year-old girl. At the communicable disease hospital, I nursed a man from Flin Flon (northern Manitoba). He had been flown to Winnipeg, as the polio vaccine wasn't available in Flin Flon yet.

I remember working at the children's hospital with a young Indigenous boy from northern Manitoba who had been living with a wolf. They believed that the boy had suckled the wolf and so was able to stay alive. He had tuberculosis (TB) of the spine. He was a favourite with the nurses. There were still several TB patients. Antibiotics, rest, and fresh air seemed to help them recuperate.

Our hospital had a wing for unmarried girls. To offset their keep, they worked in the laundry and kitchen. I worried that I might end up meeting someone I knew there. Sure enough, the first time I was placed in maternity, there was someone I knew. She had gone to the same school as me. I was just a junior at the time, and I said to the charge nurse, "I can't go in there because I know that girl." I got straightened out fast and looked after this girl for several days. As it turned out, I was the one who was embarrassed. The girl's baby was adopted by her parents.

As students, we were paid ten dollars a month in coupons. Part of that was for sanitary pads and the rest we spent in the "tuck" shop at the hospital. Usually the rest was spent there on hygiene products and chocolate bars.

Throughout the three years, we got the theory components. By the time we were finished training, we were able to: administer medication; do dressings, ostomy care, foot care, suctioning, tracheostomy care, continuous bladder irrigations, catheterizations and injections; set up and run intravenous lines; manage feeding tubes; carry out isolation technique; and do documentation, as well as other things.

After the three years of training, we wrote our RN exams at the University of Manitoba. Throughout our training, we worked hard without pay or much time off. We did come out with pride in what we could do. We had a good work ethic instilled in us. Our uniforms were white and caps were still worn. You could identify where someone trained by the shape and style of the cap they wore.

When I left training, there wasn't a department in the hospital that I couldn't either work in or take charge of. Surgery was my love. I applied and got an operating room position in a small town. I was on call twenty-four hours a day. For that I got $2,025 a year. The twenty-five dollars was for being on call. One of my nursing arts instructors told me that I was lucky—when she graduated, she made twenty-five cents an hour.

Very Strong Hands
Rita L.'s Story

I graduated from St Michael's Hospital in Toronto with my registered nurse credentials in 1959. I worked in the hospital after graduation. That hospital was one of the only ones in the city, other than the Jewish hospital, that served kosher food, so we got a fair number of Jewish patients there.

I was the night supervisor, and every night around 9 p.m. I would receive a phone call from a Mr. M., who would make a fuss at bedtime that his nurse on duty was not giving him a satisfactory back rub. The bedtime routine was as follows:

- Give patient p.m. medications.
- Wash teeth, and if dentures, soak in saline.

- Give good back rub.
- Straighten bedclothes.
- Do you wish to have drapes closed or open?
- Good night and leave.

One evening, Mr. M. was especially demanding, so I thought I would give it a try. "Good evening, sir. Did you have a good day? I see the doctor came to see you."

He responded, "Yes, nurse. So what is new?"

I said, "I will give you a back rub, as the floor nurse is extremely busy with a new admission."

"Okay," he said.

"I have good strong hands. Don't worry, this will be a good rub."

I rubbed and pushed so hard he rolled out of bed. I said, "I did not want you to relax into a bowl of jelly."

Then the trouble started.
- I had to call the front office.
- Write a detailed report of the incident.
- Call the resident "on call" to get him checked out for any damage.

Meanwhile, Mr. M. was enjoying all the attention.

I said to him, "Sir, I think you had better stay with your own nurses.

"Yes," he replied. "They are very, very good."

Rita shared her story with me when she was a few months shy of her ninetieth birthday in 2020. She smiled with great pride when she showed me her hands. Interestingly, giving a back rub is not common practice in many areas of nursing today.

Nursing in the Late 1960s to Early 1970s
Brenda's Story

Brenda writes about her experiences during her training in the late 1960s and early 1970s. She also writes about how she decided on her career path and about her working experience.

In 1969, unless you were very wealthy and could afford to pay to be a doctor or lawyer, the only work for girls was as either a teacher, nurse, or secretary. I didn't want to stand in front of a classroom and teach children of any age. My mother had been a Grade One teacher for years. I didn't want to do "just paperwork" as a secretary. Sadly, in my last few years of nursing, that is mostly what I did do. So, choices being limited, I chose nursing. I didn't come to this just by the process of elimination, because I really did want to become a nurse. I wanted to help people, so I was happy when I was accepted at St. Mary's Hospital School of Nursing in Montreal. It was a well-known and respected school that used a holistic approach to care. Part of the application entailed psychological testing. You had to get at least seventy-five percent on each exam and not just fifty percent or sixty percent to pass. While there, we learned like apprentices on the job. We had a lot of classwork and, as I mentioned, we needed to do well. I believe this is the way it should be done now.

I decided in second year of training that I wanted to work in geriatrics. This was mainly because of my practical training, when I spent time at the Douglas Hospital's geriatric ward in 1971.

When I reflect on it, there were some things that were truly awful at the time. This included bath time, when people were lined up and washed in rows like cattle, some screaming in fear. When they were calmed, I enjoyed listening to their stories and finding out what I could do to make them feel more comfortable and at peace. The main incentive or reward to keep at it was the occasional smile or thank you that I got from patients. I didn't need to be a supervisor to prove I was good at my job.

I knew I didn't want to work in psychiatry because of my time spent at the Douglas Psychiatric Hospital. I found there were two kinds of workers there. There were those who cared and really wanted to help the patients. There were those who were there for the relatively easy pay for little physical work. The latter could get away with doing very little and call it "therapy." The children's ward at the hospital was awful, as they didn't know what to do with children with autism then. The main preoccupation was to prevent them from hurting themselves or others.

While at the Douglas, I remember an Inuit man who had his condition controlled with medications. They told me he couldn't be sent home to the north. I was told that because he was mentally disturbed, he would be put on an ice floe alone, and they would send him off to die. They would not believe he was cured. I also remember a young girl in her early twenties who had severe depression. They had done a partial lobectomy to "cure her." This left her almost completely unable to care for herself.

I believe the therapy for the rest of the patients was useless. There were very few drugs to use to control or manage their conditions. Treatment consisted of people sitting around in a circle and talking. I'm not sure if there was any one-to-one therapy at all. It seemed that there was practically no progress in anyone's condition.

My time in obstetrics was not very eventful except for the time I was told to "blow" in a newborn's face repeatedly to stimulate his breathing. The baby's respirations were depressed because his mother had been given Demerol at a critical point before delivery. I can't explain why I would have been instructed to do this. I guess we didn't have any pediatric oxygen masks at the time. I do know that I vowed not to take Demerol myself, no matter what stage of labour I was in.

It was so silly that, at the age of eighteen, we were expected to take turns giving "baby bath demonstrations" to mothers who already had one or more babies. We were so awkward doing it. At least, I know that I was awkward. We were all petrified of dropping the baby while trying to hold it with one hand and wash its hair with the other, all while the baby was being held over the basin of water. Of course, there was always the chance that the male babies might produce an unexpected shower of their own during this most serious demonstration.

FRONT LINE NURSING STORIES

My placement at the Children's Hospital in Montreal in 1971 brings back lots of memories. I will always remember this little seven-year-old boy in isolation. He had a brain tumour. He asked me in French, "Am I going to die?" I could only answer him, "Who told you that?" I also remember the three- or four-year-old boy whose name was Joey. He was the product of a man who raped his own daughter. The child was profoundly mentally and physically disabled. Joey couldn't see, speak, or move on his own. His legs were in traction, as both were broken. No one knew how this had happened. The only reaction one could get from him was a small smile when you said his name in his ear or placed a small radio playing soft music near his ear.

At Children's Hospital I remember a six-year-old child who bit my finger when I tried to stroke her hair through the bars of the crib. She had been abused. I knew I didn't want to work in pediatrics because of these and many other sad stories that broke my heart.

I decided that I liked the medical unit the best, as opposed to the surgical unit. This was because usually these patients stayed longer and were often older. Many of them had chronic conditions, such as heart disease, arthritis, Parkinson's, multiple sclerosis, etc. Because they were often in hospital longer, I was able to get to know them better. I would have time to get to know them fully in all aspects. I could help them in body and mind. That is why I chose to work in geriatrics and work in a nursing home. I could get to know them so much better over time.

This decision made, I started to work part-time in local nursing homes and retirement homes.

One Christmas Day, I was at the main desk in the local sixty-bed nursing home. The desk faced the sitting room. There were two toilets and a sink area in the short hall on either side leading to the sitting room. A staff member had put a lady in one of these rooms to change her soiled clothes. They did not use adult diapers or Depends in 1986 in that particular home. The staff member left her to go and get some clean clothes. I was standing at the desk, speaking to a male visitor. I looked up and the lady was walking down the short hall behind him, completely naked. She had left the bathroom on her own. The staff member had not returned with the clean clothes. I tried casually to say "excuse me for a minute" to the visitor and quickly ushered the lady back into the bathroom. I tell you, I was so upset and had words with this staff member later during the shift.

I ended up working the rest of my career at a Home for the Aged in southeastern Ontario, from 1988 until 2011, when I retired. A new building was built, and we moved into it in 2005.

In the old building there were long hallways for each wing. Many ladies would sit in an alcove area in the afternoon. There was a relative of a resident who often visited in a silver fox fur coat. One of the ladies, who wasn't more than ninety-five pounds, was a little confused but very outspoken. She had worked for many years in a local fur store. One day the visitor with the fur coat came in and passed this little resident, who shouted, "Huh, that is nothing but a cheap beaver coat." We tried to hush her, but she just kept saying it… again and again.

I was told by some of the staff about a situation that happened which was just like the movie *Weekend with Bernie*. They told me it happened in this residence before I was working there. There was no morgue in the old building, and sometimes we would put a deceased person in the chapel before the funeral director got there to pick up the body. This was so the roommate would not be upset by having the deceased person left in his or her room. Sometimes it was for other reasons. One day, some dignitaries arrived at the home for a tour. They had to move the body out of the chapel to the library, then to a storage room, then back to the chapel, etc. The body was moved to various rooms until the dignitaries finally left.

We went through the January 1998 ice storm in that old building. There was a generator that allowed us to keep some lighting on when we lost power. One cognitively impaired lady kept saying, "But why can't I watch my TV? The lights are on. I'm missing my favourite show." The lights did not work in the bathrooms, even with the generator. The staff had to take large flashlights into these areas to help residents get ready for bed. This continued for four or five days until power was restored.

In the 1970s, we still used glass bottles for IV solutions. We used glass bottles and reusable equipment for catheters and in surgery. We used glass syringes to give medications. They were all cleaned and sterilized between patients! And I remember that from 1986 to 1995, we had to apply creams and change bandages with the cheap, disposable, "one size fits all" plastic gloves like you get now in the dollar stores.

FRONT LINE NURSING STORIES

Working in Obstetrics in the 1960s to 1980s
Mary's Story

Mary likes to remember the years she worked in obstetrics from the 1960s to the 1980s. She is now a grandmother and has seen many changes over time.

I worked in obstetrics in a hospital in Ontario. During the 60s, 70s, and 80s I remember that after a baby was born, they stayed in a separate area from their mom. At the hospital where I worked, the nursery was on the same floor but in a different wing from where the mom stayed post-partum. There was a large window in the nursery where visitors came to view the babies between two and four in the afternoon and seven and eight in the evening. Other than that, the curtain to the nursery was usually pulled across the window.

Each nursery had a very large canvas apron that hung at the door. It had ten large oblong pockets to hold ten bundled babies. This was set up so that one nurse could carry ten babies out of the building to safety in case of fire. Thankfully, I never saw the apron used.

On average, mothers who had a normal vaginal delivery stayed in hospital for five days. Mothers who had C-sections stayed in hospital for seven days. The baby was brought to the mother's bedside for feeding every three to four hours. Babies were taken to their mothers in big wooden trolleys that had five compartments. The babies were swaddled in blankets, one baby to each compartment; most had a bottle of formula beside them. I can still hear them rattling down the corridors, with babies crying because they were ready to feed. The nurse always checked the baby's ankle bracelet against the mother's armband to make sure the right baby was given to the right mother.

It was thought that the mother needed to rest after the delivery. Diapers and formula were provided by the hospital. Most mothers bottle-fed their infants. Moms were given back rubs. They were provided with sanitary pads and sanitary belts. They had sitz baths and heat lamp treatment for their episiotomies. We made linseed poultices and used flatus bags to relieve the terrible gas pains after C-sections. When I had a C-section, I found so much relief and was thankful for the poultice. I believe that these were stopped because of fear patients might be burned.

When mother and baby left the hospital, they were brought by wheelchair to the front entrance, where they were taxied away by family. Most mothers took their babies home with the baby sitting on their lap in the front seat of the car. In 1979, it became law that parents had to have infant car seats. Shocking, isn't it?

From that time, things have changed quite a bit, and I believe we have gone back to the old ways of having a baby. In some ways, things are more natural and there is less intervention. Mom and baby are kept together so they can bond. Breast-feeding is done on demand; lactation consultants are available for support. Today there is less intervention for normal labour and delivery. There are no preps before delivery. There are fewer episiotomies and C-sections. Midwifery is back, and home deliveries are in vogue.

The stories by Evelyn, Shirley, Rita, Brenda, and Mary point to the changing roles of nurses as healers. The change reflects the evolution of professionalization in nursing. This is also reflected in the way education has changed. Training in the clinical setting was the gold standard for nurses in the first half of the twentieth century. This moved to more theoretical/clinical programs in colleges and university. Entry to practice (except Quebec) has moved from a two- or three-year apprentice-type training to a university degree. As this continued to happen, the roles and responsibilities of the nurses also evolved, as will be demonstrated in upcoming stories.

FRONT LINE NURSING STORIES

Vignettes in Public Health Nursing, 1970–1995
Christine Spears's Story

Christine Spears joyfully shares vignettes from her experiences as a public health nurse (PHN) from 1970 to 1995.

Baby Visits

In 1970, the city of Toronto allocated fifty per cent of its public health spending to child and maternal health. To this PHN, it meant school nursing and new baby visits. Usually the baby visits included the expected chatting with traumatized, sleep-deprived parents about feedings, weights, and general development. It was the unexpected that I remember as I look back to those visits.

My first baby visits were in Italian-Portuguese neighbourhoods south of Queen Street West near Bathurst in Toronto. There were three baby visits due on one street. All the new parents had Italian names. When I remarked to some of the more experienced nurses that I was going to check off three visits, all on one street, on the same afternoon, they nodded knowingly to each other. They didn't say a word.

Italian and Portuguese homes in the factory-class neighbourhoods were humble and spotless. The little houses were painted pink, red, turquoise, or blue with white trim and white lace curtains. This sooty area had a true facelift when these cultures moved in. All their children attended St. Mary's Secondary School and the families worshipped at St. Mary's Catholic Church, a community parish that spoke their languages and understood their ways.

Each house had a thriving garden of vegetables, while the rest of us mostly harvested our veggies from cans and frozen food bags. Their yards for their gardens were about eight square feet, but they had something planted no matter.

The front room of each house was a small space with an array of brocaded furniture covered in plastic. I suspected it was rarely used, and the plastic was there

41

to make sure it looked rarely used. It made me feel like a VIP as I was directed to sit in this room. It was a big city–type hot day. My mini-skirted thighs stuck to the plastic. I eventually knew why the other nurses had smiled. As an obvious VIP, I was expected to toast the baby with whatever beverage was offered, and it sure wasn't tea. Mostly there were homemade wines and liquors.

After visiting three such homes, yours truly staggered to the northbound Bathurst streetcar on my trek home. My roommates wondered about my job.

Next day, my colleagues said they only did one baby visit a day in that neighbourhood.

Snakes and Babies

Keeping exotic pets was just coming into vogue. Anything more exotic than a grasshopper was plenty exotic for me. One buddy at work had a plan for any baby visits where the baby owner was also a snake owner. We could visit the home, clap loudly in the baby's face, say "Oh, good startle reflex" and leave!

Child Health Centres (CHCs)

Before OHIP [Ontario's public health insurance] came in and families could have their own family doctor, we set up free baby clinics. Mothers (fathers were rarely seen in the early 1970s) could come and chat with other mothers while their children played, nursed, and slept. They could vent any parenting woes with a public health nurse, dietician, dental hygienist, or doctor. They got the latest immunizations too. That community disappeared when we canceled the CHCs. Toy libraries eventually filled the gap, and parents could commiserate again.

One time, I had to be the Santa Claus at one CHC. There is nothing quite like having a three- or four-year-old look at you, convinced that you are Santa. It was worth all the other times you had to break the news to some parents that their kids had head lice once again.

FRONT LINE NURSING STORIES

Nursing from Bathhurst Street to Spadina and Queen Street to Lake Ontario in 1970

When I started my first PHN job for the city of Toronto, it became very clear my courses at Queen's prepared me only for the academic part of public health nursing. They did not prepare me for the real-life practical aspect of public health.

The ethnic diversity was there on a grand scale. You only had to walk ten steps around the neighbourhood, and you were in a different country—Italy, Portugal, Greece, Israel, China, Ukraine, and a small slice of the British Isles in the south. Every Thursday, the public health nurses who had areas bordering mine would meet with me, and we'd do lunch at a different country's restaurant. Speaking of food, I could stop at Kensington Market on my way home and pick up cabbage rolls and latkes. I would also get chicken wings at a dollar a pound. Why did I never franchise in the 1970s?

As a public health nurse, I was required in those days to wear a skirt or a coordinated pantsuit. Absolutely no sandals or open midriffs were allowed for fear of losing our licences. Some of the older nurses even wore little hats. We all carried the famous black bag. It held enough supplies for our visits and recording. They were heavy. When you see a retired PHN from that era, she probably has one shoulder lower than the other.

Nursing documentation was just as crucial but all done manually. Complex patient charts were the size of a copy of *Gone with the Wind*. A whole family history was contained in one chart. There were none of the high-falutin computer manoeuvres of today.

Handling phone calls for your team was a weekly experience for each of us while the rest of the team was out visiting young babies and old tuberculosis clients, hopefully not in the same house.

There were two calls I will never forget, even though they happened twenty to forty years ago. One was the man who called to say his pills got mixed up and did it matter if he got his German shepherd's digoxin. After establishing he weighed much more than his dog, I felt a little easier. However, I warned him not to let his dog get his!

The second call happened over forty years ago. As a very new PHN, I laughed first but was then struck with completely different feelings. A woman, Irma (not her real name), called and was saying to me, "You have to help me—I've been beaten and I'm black and blue all over." I madly wrote a note and passed it to a colleague to get ready to call police on another line. Then I heard a man's voice in the background.

I said, "Irma, my God, is he still there?"

She said, "Yes."

"How long has he been there?" I whispered, thinking the beating was still going on and maybe the police could catch him.

She said, "Twenty-two years."

I stifled a laugh, as does everyone at first when I tell this story—like, who would put up with this for twenty-two years? Then the poignancy hit. As I learned more about public health nursing and domestic abuse, I realized Irma's story is the story of many women, even today.

Mid-1970s College Program
Sharon M.'s Story

In the mid-1970s, I applied to the local hospital to become a registered nurse after a short and unsatisfying attempt at a teaching career. At that time, I felt I had two choices: either be a teacher or a nurse. My family was on welfare for a long time, so money was scarce. Unfortunately, the hospital-based RN program had closed its doors in Quebec. It was no longer being offered. The nursing program was now at the local college. I was disappointed but saved my money to put myself through the program.

There was much criticism about hospital- versus college-educated nurses. Hospital nurses certainly had the advantage of working in the summers and getting experience with different populations of patients. They were expected to work and not get paid. They came out with hands-on experience. In the college program, the students had their summers off and could work. Being in college, I was able to take advantage of time away and could work to pay for my courses. Each summer, I had three months to work anywhere but nursing. This is what I did. I was a decent waitress. I travelled and worked across Canada at different resorts and hotels. With a wage plus tips, I was able to save and pay my way through school. I had a very supportive mom who encouraged me to travel. Growing up, I often looked at my mom and made a promise to myself that I would never be in her situation.

In my second year of nursing, we were offered either a pediatric or obstetric practicum as our first experience. I chose pediatrics because of my supply teaching experience. I thought I would get it over with and then never have to be around a group of kids again. My expectations were incorrect! I absolutely loved my pediatric rotation. I could have easily done it again. I was a bit older than most of my classmates and thought my professor was a bit hard on me. We had to do nursing care plans and add them to our patients' charts. For homework, we had to write about our actions, discuss the patient's emotions and progress, compare lab values, etc. If something was abnormal, we had to indicate why and discuss what was happening within the illness context. We had to include the psychological and social aspects of patient care. I spent hours writing and rewriting these plans. Unfortunately, this was before the age of computers.

At times, I was not the ideal nurse. I had one patient who was from the Northwest Territories. He was having all kinds of procedures done, and no one was visiting him. He had syndactyly (webbing) of his hands and feet. He spoke no English and was obviously terrified. As his nurse, I decided that he needed to be a child and play. We sat down in the hallway and played Frisbee. It seemed to me that this was very much frowned on by more professional nurses. I was a student nurse, from the college program, so "what did I know?" This little patient smiled, laughed, and engaged with me. Even today, I can still picture his sweet little face. We did not have computers, cellphones, or tablets at the time. It was sad because if we did have them, this child could have at least seen his family.

When I did my medical/surgical rotation, my patient was an "older" lady. (I certainly would not think of her as "older" now that I am seventy.) This patient had uterine cancer. Her belly was huge, smelly, and filled with pustules. In order to provide service, I applied two masks. On the inside mask I dropped some mouthwash. This was so I could breathe in the mouthwash and not the foul odour. I proceeded to do whatever needed to be done, all the while speaking with my patient without gagging. At the end, my patient had tears rolling down her face. I inquired why and she stated that I was the first nurse not to gag or vomit while doing her care. She told me that she felt like such a "freak." I was so proud that I could update her nursing care plan that day.

When I graduated in 1974, I felt like Mary Tyler Moore, throwing her hat into the air. I decided I wanted to do outpost nursing and flew to Newfoundland. I was there for three days and decided that I was tired of waiting for planes to receive the "all clear" to fly north. Instead of flying north, I flew west back to Montreal and applied to Montreal Children's Hospital. I wanted to work on a floor that was somewhat familiar to me, but… there were no positions. I was offered intensive care, which I declined. I did not think I had enough experience to start off my career in that area. Human resources mentioned something about emergency, and I immediately said YES! I was very blessed to work with such an amazing group of nurses and physicians there. I had finally found my "calling." I learned so much from these very compassionate and experienced nurses. I will always be so grateful.

Vancouver's Downtown Eastside 1980s
Eloise's Story

This goes back to when I was about twenty-five years old and working in public health—some thirty-five years ago. I had to go see a client in the Downtown Eastside of Vancouver. The patient lived in a rooming house there. This isn't considered the best part of Vancouver, as it is an area where a lot of sex workers and drug addicts live and hang out. Typically, if we were going somewhere that we had concerns about, it was recommended that we take another nurse with us. I had been to the downtown core once before when I learned how to take the blood samples. There was a needle exchange program where addicts could come in and get clean needles and get tested for HIV. I had an uneasy feeling then.

I went to the rooming house that day with another public health nurse who worked in the downtown core. That was her district. She was very familiar with the area and said many of the places had people living in the hallways of buildings. She agreed it might not be safe for me to go in there alone. Looking back, she could probably sense my apprehension. She was an older, experienced nurse. I felt comfortable going there with her.

I was working on a special project related to cholesterol levels. We had to take cholesterol levels and take blood samples from people. We had to ask different questions about their diet and blood pressure and take their blood samples. I had to go to this rooming house where the patient lived. The patient was one of the people who I was doing a random blood sample on. I called ahead to say I was planning to visit. The patient said that was fine with him. I didn't recognize the area from the address and phone number.

As soon as we walked into the rooming house, there was an odour of feces, urine, and vomit. The stench was overpowering. I felt sick to my stomach. I saw these scary-looking homeless people and they looked foreign to me. It wasn't something I was used to seeing. I tried not to touch anything or panic. The other nurse was fine, as this wasn't something new to her. This was the district where she worked regularly.

We went into the house and went into this scantily furnished room. There was a dresser and a bed in the room. A man was sitting on the side of the bed. He had long hair. He was generally unkempt, unshaven, was missing teeth, and smelled of smoke.

I was doing my questionnaire, and he was answering. He agreed that I could take his blood. He showed me where I could take the blood and told me where to get the best veins. It was clear to him as he had many tracks there. He was very cooperative. He guided me. His veins were large. I had never seen track marks before. I felt astonished. This wasn't something I saw when growing up. I thought, *Oh my God. I've never seen anything like this before*.

As we were walking out, I could hear something behind me. It was this man with a dildo in his hand, running after us. The other nurse said, "Let's get out of here." I took off like a rocket.

I told her I didn't think I could ever work down there. She said, "Oh, well… you get used to it." She didn't sound worried at all. There was a comfort in her voice.

But it didn't matter what she said. I just knew it wasn't something I wanted to do. After that I realized that this was my bias—the people who are homeless, drug addicts, etc. I felt unsafe and recognized this type of work would not be for me. Looking back, I realize that because they are homeless and drug addicts, it doesn't make them bad people. My biases came out that day and I got to understand myself better. I didn't trust these people. I felt fearful. What if they cornered me and I couldn't get out? It was a day I will never forget.

I also won't forget the other experienced nurse. I was astonished by how she went about her job so comfortably and not at all threatened by the environment we had left. For her, it was just another day. She knew when to get out of the situation and that basically most of these people were harmless.

That was in the 1980s. If it was today, I think I would still have a fear, but now I think I would have a better sense of when to leave. If I had been alone, I would have walked in and walked out. Or perhaps I would not have gone past the smell. Being in the area and having this experience opened my eyes to the number of people with drug problems and to the homeless population.

Eloise was able to identify her fears and to closely examine herself and what happened. She was very honest with herself. This was not an area of work or a population where she could envision herself providing support.

FRONT LINE NURSING STORIES

Most Memorable Nursing Experience 1990s
Betty's Story

A forty-four-year career in nursing, which included working in a hospital, doctors' offices, Victoria Order of Nursing (home visiting), and public health, has left me with a variety of memorable experiences. One stands out as the most significant for me. Although I had accumulated many courses to maintain my currency in nursing, I decided to attend Ryerson Polytechnic University full-time in 1992 to obtain a bachelor of science in nursing. My clinical experience was at a drop-in centre for people on the street in downtown Toronto.

Coming from a small town, and from a life in which the issues these patients dealt with were foreign to me personally, I felt a little out of my element. Yet I persevered, and it remains my most memorable experience in nursing. I was partnered with an addiction counsellor who had a background in public health nursing. Up to 120 people came through the doors of the drop-in centre daily, often with mental health and addiction issues and requiring everything from the necessities of life, such as housing and food, medical attention, and counselling.

There was a sense of busyness and sometimes urgency in the drop-in, combined with the need to provide a safe environment, even while weapons and drugs were part of street life. We removed sutures from a husband and wife who had both been assaulted and robbed while sleeping on the street. A teen Indigenous couple required formula for their new baby. A senior who lived under a bridge came to the shelter for food and companionship. He preferred sleeping outside because he thought it was safer. He talked about his time as a prisoner of war in World War II. Many of the clients we counselled were young, single men who used substances to cope with their mental health issues and/or a lack of connection with their family or community.

Along with my preceptor, I attended community meetings, such as a working group of street nurses, public health nurses, and other community partners who were concerned about the increase in tuberculosis among the homeless population. The advocacy and support provided by these community partners was fearless and exemplary.

Although I provided information sessions in the drop-in as well as other supports, I was the one who benefited the most. My most enduring memory is that I met some of the most interesting, intelligent, sensitive, dignified, albeit challenging people, who seemed to exude a worldliness that reflected having lived through experiences I could only imagine. Their issues were often multiple and complicated. It was a privilege to have this experience. It helped me develop compassion and an insight into what it's like to live on the street and to have learned what true advocacy is all about from the street nurses who worked in downtown Toronto.

In contrast to Eloise, Betty found the experience of working with homeless people to be memorable and rewarding. As professionals, we all have our own levels of comfort and discomfort with the work we do and the people we support. It is important that we recognize our biases in order to be able to perform at a high level. Eloise was afraid of homeless street culture. To her credit, she was able to recognize this and move on to an area of nursing where she could be most effective.

I Ain't No Florence Nightingale
Sharon's Story

When I was in Grade Seven, one of our assignments was to write an essay on the topic, "What do you want to do with the rest of your life?" At the time, I was confident that I wanted to be a nurse. I can't remember exactly why I wanted this. I do know that I was confident about it. There were a lot of other considerations throughout high school, but I kept going back to nursing.

I went to Laurentian University and graduated with my nursing degree in 1987. When I was there, people around me were doing their computer science degree. I am a whiz at computers. This one guy asked me, "Why nursing?" I said to him," I'm a people person and I want to talk to and interact with people. I don't want to work with computers." I said this not knowing that all these years later, the computer would be such a big part of my work. At the time, it was important for me to be with people. As I said, I am a people person.

I think nursing is such a diverse profession. There are a lot of different careers within nursing. It is transferrable, and you can travel the world and work in different places. You can do a lot of different things as a nurse. Some people see it as a calling, a passion, or vocation. I don't think of it that way. I tell people, "I ain't no Florence Nightingale." I need to be paid a decent salary for the work I do. I have compassion. I have empathy. I don't work for free. There are times, with all the extra unpaid hours, I feel I do work for free. To me, you are sympathetic and stuff, and as a nursing professional you are respected but not appreciated from a financial standpoint. The expectations are high. It is predominately a female profession in North America. I believe that there are consequences to that. When I graduated, I think there was one male in my graduating class.

I Am Not Your Handmaiden
Kathy's Story

I graduated from nursing in April 1990. At that time, nurses still wore white—either a dress or pantsuit. No jewellery was allowed, and caps were optional. I found a job working on a surgical unit close to Toronto. This meant I had to commute from cottage country, which involved at least an hour's drive either way. If I was coming home on a Friday after the day shift or going to work on Sunday for an evening shift, it meant potentially a very long trip, depending on the traffic. Historically, those times were and continue to be terrible and might require a two- to three-hour ride one way. Driving in the winter could be treacherous. A snowstorm, accident, pileup, or bad weather on the 400 [highway] would have dire consequences for travel time. Several of us nurses were commuting from in and around the area where I lived and decided to carpool. We shared the driving and the expense and had some great camaraderie.

I was glad I had found a job right away after graduating, as some of my classmates decided to take the summer off. When they ended up applying for positions in the fall, jobs were few and far between. This was during the Mike Harris years [Harris was premier of Ontario from 1995 to 2002], and his Conservative government had cut jobs and decimated so many nursing positions. Many of my classmates ended up going to the States to work.

It didn't stop there. The surgical unit where I worked was closed. I was displaced to the coronary care unit (CCU) in the same hospital. I was supposed to be grateful, as there were many job losses. The people that I carpooled with to the hospital were also displaced to other units.

In the CCU, the nurse in charge was old-school, trained in the United Kingdom. She had a tough tone. She ran the unit like it was the military. She told you what to do and you did it. Some of us who travelled together and worked on the same unit wanted to be on the same shift, if possible, so we could travel together. There was no discussion. She did not approve. She was worried about all of us being late at the same time should there be trouble on our trip to get to work.

When I worked in CCU, we did twelve-hour shifts. I remember a couple of times how unsafe it was when I was driving home alone. One time, I had worked a couple of night shifts in a row. Driving home, the sun was shining so brightly, it was hard to see and hard to keep my eyes open. Another time, after doing my stint of three overnight twelve-hour shifts, I was driving home and woke up to find I had moved three lanes over from where I was supposed to be. I woke up just in time. I pulled over to the side of the road and slept for an hour until I thought I would be better able to manage it.

I remember a couple of encounters that I would like to share. One is when I was working in the CCU unit. I had worked three twelve-hour night shifts in a row. It was busy, as usual. On the last night there was a code, and the patient died at about six a.m. It was past seven a.m. and I was trying to finish my charting. I was charting on the lady who had died. The area where I was working had a small desk with a few chairs. The nurse starting the day shift was sitting beside me. The cardiologist arrived at the unit. The nurse beside me looked at me and said, "The doctor is here. Stand up and give him your chair."

As abruptly as she said that, I turned and told her, "I am finishing my charting so I can go home, and he can get his own chair." The doctor was within earshot. She was aghast that I had replied to her this way. I guess she thought I had not shown him the respect they were accustomed to giving him. There was an expectation and culture here, and I wasn't buying into it. She then got up and gave him her chair and her pen. (This doctor had a habit of asking the nurses for the use of their pen and stethoscope when he arrived on the unit.) He did not seem upset by my response, but the nurse certainly was seething. I expected to be reprimanded at some point, but I never heard anything more.

There was another physician, a diabetic specialist, who often came to the unit to see patients. He was a big, rotund guy and he walked around with a pack of cigarettes sticking out of his lab coat pocket and sucking on candy. However, he expected his patients to watch their own blood sugars, and if they were smokers, he expected them to stop. Rather hypocritical, don't you think? He would arrive on the unit and expect the nurses to trail behind him with the charts. He never looked anything up. He expected the nurses to know the blood sugars and lab values off the top of their head. He expected the nurses to provide him with an updated report on all his patients. When he made his rounds, he would give orders for treatment and expect the nurse to update the Physician Order Sheet with them.

Just to be clear, these types of expectations and attitudes were not one-offs. It was a culture that truly existed at the time.

After my first baby and maternity leave, I changed jobs to be closer to home. It was around 1992. I worked in a jail. The physician there had ordered a medication and I thought that the dosage was too high. I called the pharmacy and spoke with the pharmacist and reviewed it. The pharmacist agreed with me. She thought it was too high and out of therapeutic range. I then called the physician who had ordered it and mentioned that I had discussed the dosage with the pharmacist and we both thought it was too high.

Well… this doctor screamed and yelled at me over the phone for a good five minutes. He tore a strip off me and berated me. He told me it wasn't my place to question him as he was the doctor. He listed the reasons why he was correct, and he gave me all his credentials. He was livid. I think, perhaps, I had threatened his authority. The phone shouting went on and on. He finished by saying, "… and that is why I am the doctor and not you." I had a concern and felt a responsibility for the welfare of the patient. I am a professional and I felt I needed to follow up. I ended up giving the medication as prescribed, but I made sure to document my concerns in the file and the measures I had taken to manage any risks. It ended up that the patient was fine. I felt better to have done my due diligence.

Over the past few years, although I have not worked in the acute care (hospital) setting, I have had a lot of exposure to it. It is now 2020 and I have seen changes. I have twin boys who have special needs. One of them also had cancer and significant medical needs. He recently passed away. This meant that I spent a lot of time as a parent with my son in the hospital setting. Now many doctors introduce themselves by their first name, get their own equipment and charts and dressing supplies, work more as a team, tend to respect the opinions of nurses and recognize the knowledge and skills of the nurses. I noticed doctors have a different attitude toward the nurses, patients, and their families, and that there is not that same dictatorial attitude and dismissal of discussion.

I graduated in the diploma program and ended up going back to school to do my bachelor of psychology degree. I did it from 1998 till 2005 part-time. At the same time, I did do some nursing (not full-time) and raised a daughter and twins. I did the psychology degree more to reach a life goal than a nursing goal. Having the added education paved the way for me to obtain my job in the community. Usually, in the community, they required a degree as well as the nursing diploma. This was before the minimum entry to practice.

I have worked for thirty years in nursing, sometimes casual or part-time, and now in the community full-time. The most important thing I have learned from my experience is that nurses need to trust their instincts. Nurses need to stand up for themselves and their patients. When you think something isn't right, listen to your gut. Trust your training, education, and experience. Don't let yourself be intimidated by others. We need to be advocates for our patients. We also need to be advocates for ourselves.

Over time, the requirement for entry into the profession became more demanding. The curriculum, knowledge base, and skills that were needed continued to expand, along with the nurse's role and responsibilities. The relationship between nurses and doctors and other health professionals also changed. In her story, Kathy describes challenging the traditional power imbalance between the nurse and the physician. At that time, it was not an easy thing to do. This challenge might have led to a reprimand or possibly a dismissal if it had happened twenty years earlier, in the 1970s or 1980s.

When We Meet
Amy's Story

I graduated from nursing with my BScN in 2004. When I finished high school, I attended the University of Guelph (1997–2000). It was here that I completed my bachelor of arts degree. During my studies at Guelph, I became more and more interested in applied social science and, in my third year, human anatomy. It was during 1999–2000, once I completed my undergrad, that I decided to apply to nursing. I moved back home to live. I soon discovered that I was accepted into nursing; however, there were no spots left in the Registered Nursing (RN) Program. An option at the time was to alternatively enter the Registered Practical Nursing (RPN) Program, which was nine months in length. From this program, I could apply and bridge into the second year of the RN program. So this is what I did. It was a collaborative program between Georgian College and York University. Having the RPN designation allowed me to work while I was studying for my degree, which really was an asset when I reflect. I did year two at Georgian and the other two years at York. The four-year program included practical experience in long-term care, working with children, and rotations in mental health, obstetrics, and public and community health.

When I reflect on my academic journey to becoming an RN, I had a few personal challenges that I was living with during that time. Particularly in my third year, I was challenged by feeling quite depressed. My marks were never an issue. I was a strong student, academically. But what I came to appreciate was that I was still processing the grief from the loss of my sister, who had died a few years before. I reached out to some of my professors and shared with them what my personal challenges were. In my final year of school, after communicating with my professors, I found them to be very supportive. They were nurses and they were teachers and they listened to me and were extremely compassionate. This has always stuck with me. Not only were they teaching their students the art of caring, but they too were applying this "art" to their students. They connected with me and my circumstance. They considered my lived experience. They were human. It really made a difference for me. With their support and awareness, I went on to successfully complete my studies and achieved my goal to become an RN with a BScN.

I feel it is important to mention that the grief and trauma that I was still processing years after the death of my sister was a valuable underpinning to who I was as a student. When I reflect now, I know that my personal experience with the death of my sister made me more empathetic to patients and families who had experienced this type of loss. Or just loss in general, really. It might be the loss that comes with the diagnosis of diabetes. It could be the grief that comes with losing a newborn or having a stillbirth. It might be a trauma that can take place in an obstetrical emergency, or even the trauma or loss that can come with a person living with Alzheimer's. It is the loss not only for the patient, but for their family as well.

4. Relationships

"Too often we underestimate the power of a touch, a smile, a kind word, a listening ear, an honest compliment, the smallest act of caring, all of which have the potential to turn a life around."
– Leo Buscaglia

Relationships can be very complex. Each of us has our own intrapersonal dynamic going on while interacting with others. The relationship we have with ourselves is determined by our values, beliefs, culture, and past experiences with people, events, and environment. As individuals, we all have our own personal baggage that affects who we are and determines our comfort or lack of comfort with ourselves, others, and our external environment. It is important that the nurse's behaviour makes patients feel that the nurse is saying: "I am here to help you in any way I can. How can I help?"

As we know from our own life experiences, relationships are important for our health and well-being. Often, good relationships produce welcome outcomes. Poor relationships usually produce stress, anxiety, and unwanted outcomes. Nursing is largely about relationships. In order to do our jobs, we need to interact with the patients we work with, and we need to connect with them to maximize the healing process. Nurses need to be cognizant of their own biases and personal "baggage," as these can become barriers to the relationships we need to build.

MARIAN FACCIOLO

The Fish Hut
Tracy's Story

I was a visiting nurse in a rural area, near a lake where they did fish hut rentals. They kept the huts in the parking lot until they were rented, so there was a parking lot full of fish huts. I had a gentleman who I visited who lived in a twelve-by-twelve fish hut with his wife. They had a hot plate, a mini-fridge, and beds. They had lived there for quite a while. They stuffed the hole [in the floor of the hut] with blankets and had a space heater to keep them warm. It was winter when I started to visit. He had a diabetic foot ulcer, and I visited him to change the dressing on his foot.

The man had a white rat named Fergus, who he told me was a member of his family. When they moved to the hut, Fergus moved with them. I was expected to treat him like part of their family. This was made clear to me at the first visit. There was a routine that I had when I made my visit there. This entailed me feeding Fergus mini marshmallows. He was in a cage, and I did not have to touch him or anything. His feeding was part of the routine. It was very important that this routine be followed. "Hi, Mr. and Mrs. G. and Fergus." Then, "Fergus, here is your food."

The patient's foot did eventually heal, even living in these conditions. It took a long time to happen. The patient did go for his treatments, and the wounds were cared for between my visits. The man didn't want to have his foot amputated.

I was never very fond of Fergus, but my feeding was part of the routine. The man had a cellphone, but it often didn't work. It wasn't a difficult visit, although I was a bit worried the first day. I think the man knew the area well, but his mobility was limited because of his ulcers and chronic condition. He didn't use the fish hut for fishing that year.

In this story, Tracy is surprised by the environment the couple is living in and by the focal point being their pet. She understands that she must not let her feelings about Fergus get in the way of helping this man heal his wound.

FRONT LINE NURSING STORIES

Experience with Snakes
Eloise's Story

The assessments and reassessments that Eloise mentions in the next story, are also mentioned by many other nurses. These areas include: a patient's physical, mental, emotional, cognitive, and support systems as well as information about the diagnosis, prognosis and medical status. Assessments are used to develop a personalized care plan with the patient/family.

I was working as a case manager for a community agency that had developed a model of care that was broken down into programs that included the "regular program" and the "complex program." As a "complex case manager," my role included working with patients with brain injuries.

One of the case managers told me she wanted to transfer a client to me. She told me the patient had been in a car accident and, as a result, had a brain injury. The patient ended up with physical and cognitive deficits, including speech problems. Included in the background information about this patient was that she used to run a travelling reptile show. This had ended, but she still had some animals in her home. This included a python, tarantulas in cages, and a parakeet perched on a shelf. When informed of this, I could only focus on the python. I admit that I am terrified of snakes.

There was no reason for me to go out immediately to see this patient. I consoled myself with the thought that I would not have to go out and reassess her for another six months. So I told myself, "All right, I will deal with it then."

No sooner was she on my caseload than I got an update: the lady had gone to hospital because of a vicious attack on her hand. The python had bitten her while she was handling it. There were torn tendons and ligaments. She required extensive surgery. The next update was that she had been treated and was returning home. The report noted that the python was gone. The patient required nursing for dressing changes and continuation of treatment related to her brain injury. Her six-month review was now due. I needed to make a home visit.

As I walked into the house, the first thing I saw was cages full of snakes. The snakes were five feet long and very skinny. I tried to settle myself and talked to myself to calm myself down. I couldn't run out, as she would think I was crazy. After all, the snakes were in cages. I decided that I wouldn't look at them. I sat on the couch and noticed that on the other side of me were the tarantulas in cages and the bird. The bird got excited with my being there, so my patient put it in another room.

The husband was there too. The lady had speech problems related to her brain injury, so it was hard to understand what she was saying. Our assessments were very thorough and took a long time to complete, even at the best of times. I was a mess and felt very nervous and vulnerable. I kept thinking of the python. The other snakes were right there in my full view. It was difficult to keep my eyes off them, no matter how hard I tried. I felt uneasy. I tried to settle myself by focusing on my patient and not looking at the snakes.

While I was sitting on the couch, I could feel something at my feet. I told myself it was just my imagination. I felt it again, but once again settled myself. I felt it again. I became very anxious. This time I jumped up off the couch in a panic and screeched. Out from under the couch came a huge turtle. It was a foot long. Her husband tried to reassure me. He told me it was the only animal that was loose in the house. By this time I knew I couldn't continue and quickly finished my visit and left. I kept thinking, *I have to get out of here.* My last thought as I was leaving was, *I don't know if I can ever go back there.*

Over the next few days, I started to worry about having to go back and reassess her. I went home and started having dreams about snakes. The dreams were quite vivid. In fact, they were nightmares. Snakes were everywhere. They were after me. In my dream, I found myself jumping up off the couch in a panic, brushing my body to rid myself of the reptiles as they crawled all over me. I would awake breathless, sweaty, and panicky.

I talked with another case manager on my team and asked if she was fearful of snakes. This case manager would do anything to help me. She said she didn't really like snakes, but they didn't bother her that much. I just couldn't go back to the home of the patient with the snakes. I was fearful to tell the patient and her husband about it. I guess I didn't want to be embarrassed. I didn't want them to feel bad, either. I thought I should have been able to manage the situation. After all, the snakes were in cages. Later, I thought maybe I could have asked them to do the interview in another room. I kept telling myself, "I can do this… I can do this." I felt that I should have been able to do it, especially since the snakes were in a cage.

You know, when I think of it, I know why I was so afraid. I had seen garter snakes when growing up. When I was in Grade Nine, a classmate of mine said, "Eloise, do you want to see what I have?" Before I could answer, he pulled a snake from his pocket. It was only a garter snake, but I jerked back and screamed.

After recess, we went to French class. The French teacher was very strict, she didn't put up with any nonsense. This same guy asked me to throw something in the waste basket. When I finally did this for him, I could see something move in the can. Once again, I screamed out. The French teacher got mad at me, but I said, "No, there is something in the can." Sure enough, it was the garter snake. Since then, my relationship with snakes hasn't been the same. If I'm out walking in the woods, I'm cautious and look around, especially if there is tall grass. If something moves, I run. I don't think that I will be able to take care of anyone again with snakes in the home. I think I will have to refuse.

Eloise wants to be able to work with this patient and family. She thinks long and hard about it and decides what she must do. The limitations are enhanced by the environment in which she must provide service. Although this story is somewhat humorous, it also underlines the impact of life experiences. Eloise's childhood experience with a garter snake had a significant impact on her ability to engage in a therapeutic nursing experience.

MARIAN FACCIOLO

When Can We Meet?
Robin's Story

As a visiting nurse out in the community, you really must be prepared for just about anything. You are on your own. You are independent and you must learn quickly how to deal with people... and their pets. As an animal lover myself, it never bothered me that the odd patient would not follow protocol and lock up their animals. Often, the fact that I loved their animals so much made for a good connection with the patient. I came to learn that if I were in the good books with the pets, I would also win over the hearts of their doting owners. One day, though, I think it went a little too far.

I was going to see a patient I had not met before. When I had made my call to her the previous night to advise her about what time she could expect to have her visit, she made it clear she was not happy to be having someone "new" to her. As she realized she would not be having her regular nurse, the tone in her voice began to have the quality of someone who was tasting a cheap wine: initially joyful, but bitter upon the finish. She reluctantly agreed for me to see her at my preferred time, and I tried to stay hopeful that she would accept me.

I set out that morning as I usually did, finally arriving at the patient's home. It was a very long jaunt. Much longer than I had expected. Her house was down a long and winding road, and at one point, I thought it led nowhere. As I was trying to make my way to her, I also realized I was not going to make our agreed-upon time. My heart started to pound. She was not happy to begin with, so I was sure the fact that I had miscalculated my travel time, which was making me late, would only add to the patient's existing perception that I was going to be less than adequate.

As I pulled into her laneway thinking that this was going to be a very uneasy visit and that I would have to try to make it as quick as possible, I was delighted to see that she had a dog. A lovely black lab. A beautiful older dog, in great shape, with what looked like a new collar with a shiny, new tag. In my mind, this meant that she cared deeply for this dog.

My anxiety melted away as the dog started dancing around my car, as excited to see me as I was to meet him. *This is my way in,* I said to myself. I looked at the house and was delighted to see the patient watching anxiously out a front window. I would have made a fuss over the dog to begin with, but the fact that I could use this opportunity to my advantage was the icing on the cake.

I made an affectionate scene over the wonderful pooch. I immediately created a bond with him, and the connection was undeniable. Having a lab, myself, I was very comfortable with this breed, and I was sure to make that obvious as my patient kept a watchful eye. I climbed the stairs to the front porch, a smile adorning my face, as I knew I had now won over this patient. My new friend was trailing on my heels, smiling and dancing around as though he fully approved of this new person who had come to care for his master.

I knocked on the door. A few seconds later, my patient answered, but instead of being met with a smile as she realized any friend of her dog was a friend of hers, I was greeted with scorn and a harsh look. I pretended not to notice this continuation of her dismay and said in a very cheerful voice, as the dog barged into the house and began running around, "I am so glad you have a dog. He is so lovely! What is his name?"

The look on her face as the dog ran around the house uncontrollably told me something was not quite right. When she said, in a raised and infuriated tone, "That's NOT my dog," I must have had a very confused look on my face. Then she started to smile and laugh and said, "I thought that was your dog! I do not have a dog. I thought you brought your dog to work."

For a few seconds, I was scared that this would only add to her disappointment in me. I repeated what she had already confirmed, just to be sure I had heard this correctly: "That is not your dog?"

"No," she replied. "I have never seen that dog before in my life."

The dog at this point was going crazy in her house. Running around, grabbing pillows off her couch, jumping on the couch, and acting as if he had never had human friends before. He was clearly enjoying himself a bit too much. I was jolted back to the reality of the scenario and called to the dog. He took this as his "play time" and started to run toward us as though he was going to let us catch him, but then at the last minute he would zig around us. This game of cat and mouse continued. After a few minutes, the patient and I decided to give it a break. There was no way this dog was going to let us catch him while he thought we were participating in his exuberance.

I asked the patient to walk away and ignore him, and I did the same. I turned my back to the dog, opened the front door and ran out of the house like a crazy woman, yelling, "Come on boy, come on, let's go play." I jumped off the deck, making myself seem more playful than I was really feeling at that moment. The dog ran out of the house to follow me, excited to have someone join him in his free time. I doubled back into the house as quickly as I had left it and closed the door behind me, locking the intruder outside, looking at the door. He had an expression of defeat as he turned and walked up the laneway.

I felt bad for him, but when I turned around and saw my patient staring at me with crossed arms, I was fully expecting her to ask me to leave. Instead, she said, "As I was watching you with the dog out my window, I was asking myself, why on Earth would she bring her dog to someone's house with her?" Then she started to laugh. It was a full belly laugh, and I had to join in.

After we got ourselves under control, I was able to complete my visit and conduct her medical care as planned. We shared many laughs about what had just happened. I left her home with a true smile on my face. The dog was nowhere to be seen. He had probably moved on to the next house to brighten someone else's day!

Robin loves dogs and she understands relationship building. This turned out to be a comedy of errors that ended up with a positive result.

Food for Care
Mary's Story

I was scheduled to work the eleven p.m. to seven a.m. overnight shift in a private home in the community. The patient was a sixty-year-old lady who needed palliative care. I knocked on the door and was met by the patient's husband and their dachshund dog. The dog growled and barked at me. Until then, I had never noticed just how long a dachshund snout was, and how many sharp teeth it held in its jaws.

I was taken into the house to meet the patient. The dog settled himself on the bed beside her. The husband gave me a report on his wife and informed me that the dog always stayed with her. He told me the dog would sleep. Then the husband went to bed, leaving me with the patient and dog. Every time I touched the patient, the dog rolled up his lips and showed his large row of teeth and growled. I thought, *This is going to be a long, difficult night.* Then I noticed how chubby the dog appeared. A light bulb went off in my head and I remembered the food I had brought for myself for the shift. I took the food out of my bag. Every time I needed to touch the patient, I fed the dog. He wasn't fussy. He ate anything. It worked like a charm, all night.

In the morning, when I told the husband what I had done, he laughed. The next night when I came to work my shift, the dog greeted me enthusiastically at the door with his tail wagging while he sniffed my bag. This time, the patient's husband had a tray of dog treats beside his wife's bed, ready for me to feed the dog when needed. He did this every night shift after that.

Mary relates how she overcame obstacles to provide the nursing care that her patient needed. Palliative care for her patient included turning and positioning, mouth and skin care, toileting, administering medication for pain and comfort, and emotional support. Mary needed to get physically close in order to meet her patient's needs and provide basic nursing care.

Over time, there has been a major shift toward community nursing. The purpose of this shift is to reduce expensive hospital services but also because many people prefer to receive medical care at home. The impact of this shift on nursing has been significant on many fronts. These animal stories, although humorous, point to some potential new risks for nurses. Nurses working in hospitals have no worries about getting attacked by vicious dogs or dealing with snakes.

The increased focus on community nursing has also resulted in the need for nurses to treat medical conditions with greater acuity than ever before. There is often a lag time for medical backup in the community compared to the hospital setting, which leads to a greater need for quick problem-solving and independent decision-making.

Like-Minded Providers
Karen's Story

As a community nurse, I have had the privilege of supporting many patients and their families at the end of their lives. One patient who had an impact on me was an elderly farmer who was dying of cancer. This man lived with his two bachelor sons, who also helped run their small farm. Their household had not seen a woman's touch since the patient's wife had died many years before. Their home was a very basic farmhouse, and it had seen better days. The drive to the house was overrun with brush, and anyone venturing in needed help from the sons to navigate. The floors felt as if they were about to collapse, and the bathroom probably hadn't been cleaned in years.

Even though the sons were not educated, were not particularly comfortable with health care professionals, and were not sophisticated, they really wanted to support their father to die with dignity at home. We were able to build a team of community supports for them. Everyone involved was non-judgmental. We all became comfortable in this very neglected home. We all worked hard to ensure that this family of three men was supported in whatever manner they were comfortable. The sons trusted the visiting nurses and followed all their instructions. When it was clear that their father was within hours of dying, they asked that they be left alone with him. They wanted their father to be allowed to die in the same room that he had been born in, with his sons at his side. They may not have been a very sophisticated family, but they were certainly very wise, and they had the respect of all who were fortunate enough to be involved in their journey.

In this story we learn about a group of providers who were all on the same page in values and support for this patient and his family. Karen recounted the story with nostalgia, as if it had been a magical experience.

Adopting a Kitten
Karen's Story

I was working as a new grad in an in-patient acute psychiatry unit. One night, I admitted a very scared fifteen-year-old girl, Natalie, for treatment of depression. She was dressed all in black; her style was Goth. Black nails, black lips, black clothes—everything black. She came across as being tough, but it didn't take much scratching of the surface to learn that she was an insecure, scared girl who was looking for approval. As her primary nurse, I spent lots of time with her and thoroughly enjoyed all of it. I remember her talking at length about how uncomfortable it made her when people stared at her. This struck me as quite funny, considering her outrageous appearance, but of course I didn't laugh out loud—just an inside chuckle. We explored her motives for shocking people, and she had clear family dynamics that provided clues to this behaviour.

One day, Natalie came back from a day pass. She was close to discharge and was spending more time at home. When I walked into her room, I heard a kitten meow. Natalie pulled it out of her pocket, telling me her mother was going to put the litter down. She begged me to keep one. Since I was single, it didn't take much convincing for me to adopt this beautiful calico cat. We found a box and I hid her in the nursing station, hoping my head nurse wouldn't discover her. I am pretty sure she knew the kitty was there. She chose to look the other way for the rest of my shift.

I had that kitty for many years. She was with me when I met my future husband, got married, and had my three children. I often thought about Natalie and wondered how she was doing. A few years after acquiring my kitty, I ran into her at a festival. She looked the same but had a big smile and gave me a hug. My youngest is now the same age Natalie was when she was admitted to the psych unit. Natalie taught me that teenagers might look tough and uninterested on the exterior, but they are often scared and insecure underneath. I hope she is having a good life.

Sometimes nurses need to take some risks and unusual steps to establish relationship.

I Want My Milk
Kathryn's Story

A step-down unit is an area where patients who need closer monitoring are sent from the intensive care unit (ICU) before they go to a regular acute care ward. The nurse-to-patient ratio in the step-down unit allows patients to receive closer observation.

At one point, I had a patient in a step-down unit who enjoyed the extra attention and called for help with all sorts of things in order to get it. For example, "My pillow needs to be fluffed." "I need another blanket." "I want a snack." "Take off the blanket… " "My toe hurts… " "Turn my pillow over," etc. etc. etc.

"Mr. Needy" was stable, and I was waiting for a bed on the ward to become available in order to transfer him there. At the same time, I had a very unstable patient who was seriously ill and needed close monitoring. He was located right across from the stable but demanding patient. At one point, Mr. Needy said, "Why is he getting all the attention? What about me?"

As the unstable patient became sicker, it was apparent the interventions were not working. We had to call a code. While we called the code, Mr. Needy was yelling at the top of his lungs from across the room, "I want my milk!… I'm thirsty.… When are you bringing me my milk?"

I responded, "Please wait. I need to look after my other patient, as he is very sick."

Mr. Needy raised his voice and shouted, "I don't care. I WANT MY MILK."

The code was called on the unstable patient. The room filled with the crash cart and other medical personnel in order to save the man's life. We stabilized him and sent him to the ICU. He was critical and needed even closer monitoring. We no sooner got him stabilized than it was time for shift change.

Mr. Needy, who observed all this, still demanded his milk. I gave a report to the oncoming nurse in charge. I did not want her to have to deal with Mr. Needy's demands for milk, so before I left I went to the fridge down the hall, got a small carton of milk with a straw, and gave it to him. He did not say thank you, just replied, "Open it and put the straw in." I did this for him and said, "Good night; you will have another nurse this evening."

As I was walking out of the room, I heard him spit the milk out of his mouth and say crossly, "This milk is sour."

I left the building.

The next morning, I got a report from the night nurse and asked if Mr. Needy had been calling all night. She said, "No, he was quiet and actually pleasant." I have to say, I too found him more polite that morning. He was soon transferred to the ward, and he did not ask me for milk again.

In this story, Kathryn talks about a patient she found difficult to connect with during her busy shift. Most shifts are busy, and nurses are required to continually prioritize patients' needs. Workload can adversely affect the relationship with patients. Of course, nurses never intend for this to happen, but high workload and stress can interfere with both process and outcome. In this instance, the unstable man would have died without the medical attention he received. Consequently, "Mr. Needy" became angry with the nurse. Kathryn's heavy load didn't allow her to effectively explore what his needs really were. It is uncertain what intrapersonal things were going on with him.

Words Can Mean a Lot
Cora's Story

Mrs. S. was a seventy-two-year-old with multiple sclerosis (MS). In her younger years, before her move to our area, she had been an RN who lived in Ontario and commuted every day across the border to work in a hospital in the US. She had five children who were spread out from Halifax to London, Ontario. She did have one daughter who lived in our community, not too far from her parents. She had a terrific spouse who was devoted to her and who managed all her care.

When I first met the family, Mr. S. was scheduled for a knee replacement and wanted to discuss the options for managing his wife's care during his hospital stay and recovery period. At that time, Mrs. S. needed assistance with transfers, showers, and getting dressed. She was also dependent for meal preparation, housekeeping, laundry and shopping. She could walk very short distances with a walker, but was primarily using a scooter.

Mrs. S. could go outside and garden in the elevated flower beds that her spouse had built for her. She was able to walk her Rottweiler dog using her scooter. I observed that her posture was poor when sitting on the scooter. I recommended that she have an occupational therapist (OT) do an assessment for transfers and to discuss equipment to make it easier for her to function at home.

Mrs. S. was put on the waiting list for rising and retiring care at home, as well as for the short-stay respite list at long-term care. The hope was that this would provide support and relief for her spouse. Mrs. S. did get the support at home during Mr. S.'s recovery from surgery. The daughter who lived in the area assisted during the day as well. The OT helped the couple get funding for the purchase of both a power wheelchair and a ceiling lift to facilitate with transfers. The family arranged for a ramp from the house to the garage and a lift seat to help her get into the van.

I met with the client and her spouse every six months to reassess her needs. This was done over a period of about two and a half years. Over that time, she slowly deteriorated, and at each visit, I observed an increase in weakness and loss of physical function. I got to know the couple. They got to know me better and to feel comfortable with me.

Mrs. S. had follow-up appointments yearly at the MS clinic at Sunnybrook Hospital. This provided both the family and me with the knowledge that she had specialists to oversee her specific needs.

Mrs. S. had a history of urinary retention. She refused to consider any type of catheter. As a result, she would get frequent urinary tract infections. She was hospitalized for urosepsis and treated. There was a poor response to the antibiotics and her condition deteriorated. More than anything, she wanted to return home. Her spouse agreed to bring her home and was more than willing to help with her care. He did not have any idea what to expect. I made a home visit, and at that time Mrs. S. was having periods of unresponsiveness. I explained to her spouse that she was dying. I explained what he could expect in the next few days and what to do when she passed away. He was tearful but also grateful, because no one had explained anything to him at the hospital. I arranged for nursing visits and for a personal support worker to provide shift support during the night. Mrs. S. passed away the next day.

Over the next month, Mr. S. called me three times to thank me. He would also tell me each time about how much he missed his wife.

Mr. S. took a car trip to Halifax to see his son. On his way back, coming up Highway 400, he got a flat tire. He wasn't that far from home. He called his daughter from the roadside and told her what happened. His son-in-law said he would come and assist him. This happened at midnight. Before his son-in-law arrived, Mr. S. stepped out of the vehicle and was hit by a transport truck and killed.

About a month later, I received a phone call from the couple's daughter, asking me how she would go about donating her mom's equipment. I referred her to the MS Society loan cupboard. Then I asked how Mr. S. was doing. That is when I found out what had happened to him. His daughter told me that she thought her dad stepped in front of the truck on purpose. He was still grieving the death of his wife. I was extremely sad about the situation. They were a terrific couple. They tried to be as independent as possible. I had really connected with them. The daughter told me that my support to her parents had meant a lot to them. She told me that her dad appreciated my honesty and direction at the end of his wife's life.

Hearing her say these things made me appreciate that as nurses doing direct care, and as care case managers who assess, plan, advocate, we can and do make a difference in people's lives. It was a reminder of the positive effect our efforts can have in care we provide.

This story demonstrates how vital the connection with the nurse can be and how this can result in reciprocal benefit. Cora was able to provide ongoing support to the couple and the family. The family made the nurse feel good about her role. Cora acknowledges the personal pain she felt by being engaged and committed throughout the provision of care.

The story highlights the intense grief that can happen when a person loses a loved one. In the story, we don't know for certain whether Mr. S. did or did not step in front of the truck on purpose. We are reminded of a grieving persons vulnerability and the need for grief support.

FRONT LINE NURSING STORIES

Connection Through Music
Miae's Story

We often find common ground to bind and build our connections. Miae's story shows this quest for knowledge of her patient.

Nursing is a profession whose mission is about caring for people. People are complex beings who cannot be simply broken down to a sum of parts like an automobile can. For this reason, nursing requires us to use creative and multiple ways of knowing to engage the patient or client in the intricate, interactive relationship. This dynamic process is often more pronounced in my home visits with patients who have dementia.

For example, at my home visit with an eighty-two-year-old male patient with frontal lobe dementia and his family, I quickly realized that the routine way of collecting data was going to have to shift, because the patient was not looking at me, not communicating with me, and repetitively interrupting with remarks such as, "No, I'm not going to Swiss Chalet… no, no, no. No, I'm not going anywhere."

When I asked the client what his hobbies were, and he replied angrily, "No, I'm not going to Swiss Chalet," his brother replied for him, saying that he used to enjoy singing. Although the client continued with his repetitious negative comments, when his brother started singing the tune "Danny Boy," the patient stopped his speech and continued the song in the same key as his brother had started with, finishing the song grandiosely! All the while, the patient was not facing me.

After he finished, I applauded and genuinely told him that he had a wonderful voice. I really meant that sincerely because of my own love for good music, and the patient picked up on that. He turned and faced me for the first time, and when I offered my hand, he took it and shook it warmly and smiled. At that moment, his dementia diagnosis and my RN designation did not matter. The caring moment transcended all of that, and we briefly entered a human-to-human transaction.

As care coordinators working in the community, we are mandated by Ontario's Ministry of Health and Long-Term Care to use the RAI HC (Resident Assessment Instrument for Home Care), which is a standardized assessment tool that breaks down the client's health into several domains. In the case I described, the conventional method of using this assessment approach was not only unsuccessful, but I felt it had also impeded my initial objective, which was to connect with the client. Although the scenario illustrates only a brief time of connection between the patient and myself, I felt at that moment he understood that I valued him as an individual, and I, in turn, saw that beyond the repetitious phrases, the singer was still there. I did eventually, with family input, collect my data to complete the assessment; however, the brief experience which transcended the data collection is one that I will keep with me to ground my nursing in human caring experience.

I understand Miae's frustration about the disadvantages related to the computer assessments. Nurses do assessments and reassessments as the needs of people change. The focus has always been on the patient. However, the evolution of nursing has seen a major shift in the use of electronic assessment and charting that has significantly changed the focus, especially from the perspective of the funder and, consequently, the administrators of the health care system.

There are obvious benefits to these advances in technology. I admit, initially I was excited and optimistic about what we could do with the technology. I thought the information gathered this way could provide a focus to target prevention or to provide more appropriate resources for patients and families. I continue to see the value of technology and electronic charting to facilitate the storage, sharing and analysis of information and the potential generation of valuable research. However, developing a meaningful relationship with a patient while typing information into a laptop computer is not an easy task. It also takes a lot more time to complete the data gathering. The computerized assessments are lengthy, time-consuming, and cumbersome. They can decelerate the process of relationship building and healing.

FRONT LINE NURSING STORIES

No Time for Anne or Rosemary
Marian's Story

Many of the stories in this book show that a nurse's success in developing a good relationship with a patient and their family is important to achieve positive therapeutic outcomes.

I remember doing a home visit to complete an initial assessment. The patient, Anne, was very distraught. She had both mental health issues and dementia. She was very agitated and was unable to answer any of the questions herself. A family member was available to provide information, while the patient's anxiety continued to rise with the continuation of the questions and the family answering them. I ended up completing the assessment without the patient being present, as it was too disruptive for her. I went back later to spend some time with the patient.

I had another patient, named Rosemary, with Alzheimer's disease. Her daughter was present to provide the information. With patients who are cognitively impaired, there is still a need to get the information, and we often work with the family to obtain it. In this instance, the patient had significant cognitive impairment and behaviours and was living in a retirement home. The daughter was very upset about the situation and the amount of care she had to provide to support her dad, who was the primary caregiver. At several points during the assessment, the daughter started to cry, as she was unable to contain herself. She needed reassurance and she needed to vent. I know that I spent between two to three hours there to get the information, to comfort the daughter, and to ease the patient's discomfort with the burden of the interview.

These examples are not unusual when gathering information from certain groups of patients in the community, whether the nurse is using a computerized assessment form or not. Sometimes the patients get anxious or frustrated with the meeting. They can express their anxiety in different ways, which include different types of behaviours.

Call Me Charlie
Kathryn's Story

I recall a pleasant elderly gentleman I looked after on a busy medical ward. He had dementia but would recognize me as his nurse and looked forward to seeing me. I introduced myself initially as Kate, as this is my name. He told me that I was a nice young man and he called me "Charlie." Whenever he saw me, he called me Charlie.

After a few days passed, I decided he should be reminded of my real name again. I greeted him as always, and after he said, "Good morning, Charlie. I'm glad you're back," I told him, "Mr.—, my name is Kate. I'm a girl."

He responded with a perplexed expression and said, "How do you spell that?"

I clearly replied, "K… A… T… E."

He looked at me and repeated the same letters, then said, "Well! That's a funny way to spell Charlie."

After this, I decided to be Charlie for him, as that is who I was in his mind.

Kathryn had a good connection with this patient. She understood his disease and the limits imposed by it. "Charlie" and the patient continued to develop a rapport.

FRONT LINE NURSING STORIES

Death Looming
Marian's Story

I was in charge of a medical/surgical unit. It was the evening shift. As charge nurse, my role included passing out the medications, including the night sedation. Being in charge was considered an important role, especially for a new grad. It also meant that any issues or concerns regarding clients, staff, and doctors were my responsibility. I usually did this well, which is why I was often put in this position, even though it was only my second year of work since graduating from nursing. It felt good to be so valued.

I recall this one night. At bedtime, while doing rounds, I visited John. He was a fifty-six-year-old man who had come to hospital with a pathological fracture of his femur. He had already had the surgery required. He had also had a battery of tests. It was discovered that he had cancer. I remember that John had a wife who was supportive and who visited him regularly. Although I remember her visits, I don't remember them ever speaking to each other. This seemed strange to me.

The night that I was in charge and passing out the medications, I was aware that John knew his diagnosis. The cancer had spread. The patient knew this. When I went to his bedside with the medications, he was very quiet. He let me know that he wanted something for pain and something to sleep. After administering the medications, he just looked at me and I looked back. What could I say? What could he say? He then asked me to stay with him a while. Given the circumstances, I stayed with him. My other patients would just have to wait!

I stood by the bedside and we looked at each other in silence. He reached out to hold my hand. He gazed into my eyes for what seemed like a very long time. We just looked at each other and held hands. I didn't have much experience with death and the dying process. I did not feel hope for John. I think I was as devastated as he was with the news. He looked very sad and hopeless as he gazed at me. Was he looking for hope? I had none. Thinking back, I believe that he got comfort from my just being there with him. He was not alone. I console myself with this.

After that evening, I was off work for four days. During my time off, I thought of John often. I thought of him holding my hand, staring into my eyes and searching. Every day I wondered if he would be there when I got back.

During my trip back to the hospital, I was consumed by thoughts of John. I actually had a sick feeling about him as I made my way to the unit. Once I got to the nursing station, the first question I asked was about how John was doing. I was told that he had passed away. In one way I wasn't surprised, but on the other it seemed to happen so quickly. The news wrenched at my gut. I felt very sad. There was no time to mourn. I had to function and be strong for the shift ahead of me. I did feel sad and took my sadness home to weep there.

Whenever I think back to that time with John, I am satisfied that I was able to provide him with comfort that night we held hands.

Sometimes when I think back, I wonder if I should have expressed more hope. Maybe he was looking for that. Would he have felt my hope? I know he would eventually have died, but maybe he would have lived a little longer. That is the part I will always wonder about.

I can remember my interaction with John so well. It feels as if it happened yesterday. The patient was old enough to be my father. As a student nurse and new grad, I had experiences that reinforced my belief that I could make a difference. In this scenario, the value of touch drove home to me how every person is different, and healing occurs in so many ways. Over the years I developed more comfort and confidence dealing with death and dying. I have also come to better understand the importance of hope in the process of healing and dying.

FRONT LINE NURSING STORIES

I Feel Your Pain
Marian's Story

The following story remains alive in my memory and in my heart. The value of being present can be overlooked.

The labour and delivery unit is mostly a happy place to work. It is also an unpredictable place, as one never knows who will come into the unit next, and at what stage of labour.

We got a call at the nursing station from one of the obstetricians. His voice was tense; he certainly did not sound like his usual self. He informed me that he was sending in one of his patients who had come to his office for a visit. The patient was full term but had not felt any fetal movements for a few hours. The doctor couldn't get a fetal heartbeat. The patient was coming to the unit straight from his office for fetal monitoring and possible induction.

On arrival, she was quickly admitted. A fetal monitor was put in place. There were still no movements. Her husband joined her soon after her arrival. The obstetrician came within what seemed like minutes. Both were there for support. We started the induction as per the doctor's orders. Before too long, she was in active labour and the induction wasn't needed any more.

My shift was ending, but the patient was close to delivery, so I decided to stay to see her through this. Her husband sat at the head of the delivery table by her side. She was encouraged to push and push again and again until finally the head was crowning. She delivered a perfect baby girl. All fingers and toes were accounted for, and she was a beautiful seven-pound baby. I remember looking at this beautiful new person. I recall being surprised that her colour was still pink, as she was lifeless. No need to suction this perfect baby. No need for any gentle stimulation for a lusty cry. No cries were expected.

There was a "true knot" in the umbilical cord. A true knot is just as it says. Nutrients and oxygen pass to the baby via the umbilical cord. It is baby's lifeline. If there is a knot and it tightens, it can be dangerous. If the knot tightens enough, it can cause brain injury or fetal death for the baby.

The doctor put the baby onto mom's tummy after the birth and quickly wrapped her in a blanket for them to hold. The couple looked exhausted and overwhelmed with sadness and grief. Tears streamed down their cheeks as they held and gazed at their newborn baby in silence.

I had no words. I had only an overwhelming feeling of sadness for a life that would never be. Standing next to the couple, I looked at this perfect baby and then at her parents. As our eyes met, I felt tears run down my face. Our hearts met for one brief moment, and they knew I shared their pain. Being present for them seemed to validate their own pain the way no words could ever do.

I went home that night feeling extremely sad. Somehow I felt that I was the right person to be with them and to share in this painful event. I wondered whether I would be able to withstand any more of these painful experiences. Although there was some satisfaction with the amount of emotional support I had offered this couple, I wondered if I would one day shut down. It was a risk that I decided I would continue to take, at least for now.

Death and a Stolen Bike
Kerry's Story

This is a short but beautiful story. I did not have a whole lot to do with it. It was just the way things worked out.

I had a patient who lived in a rural area. She was in her early thirties with end-stage ovarian cancer. She had six young children, all under the age of ten, a very supportive husband, a very supportive sister and a very supportive mother. Her wish was to remain at home, despite all the kids and despite the fact they were so young. She wanted to die at home. That wish was granted. She was well supported by her family throughout her illness. It was a comfortable passing. On the night she passed away, she was surrounded by the people who she cared for most.

In my view, the way this couple dealt with the experience was precious and perfect. The kids were part of her illness from day one. They knew what was going on at their own level. All their questions were answered. They knew that Mommy would be going to heaven and she would see them all later on when they were grown up. They seemed to be okay with this. To watch them converse with their mom and dad about it was amazing. I think kids have a way of adapting. You could see that they thought: *all right, this is what is going to happen.* They accepted it.

Unfortunately, on the day after her passing, the kids got up in the morning, and one of the youngest, around four or five years of age, discovered that his bike had been stolen. At first, I couldn't believe it. This was a small rural town where everyone knew what was happening with their neighbours. It was a small community, and the people living there knew that this lady was dying. I thought, *Who would ever... ever... do such a thing? Take a child's bike. Especially knowing what this family was going through!*

That day I had gone out to the home for a reassessment visit. It was early, and I hadn't yet been notified that the mother had passed away during the night. I knew she was getting close, and I wanted it to be successful for this family, so I went over to check on things first thing in the morning. When I got there, the young boy was crying that someone had stolen his bike. He was extremely distraught. This event was taking over what had happened with his mom.

I went to him and casually said, "Honey, you know what? I bet that Mommy needed that bike to get to heaven faster. You actually helped her!"

Well, suddenly, that was the end of his tears. He was as proud as could be that he helped his mom get to heaven on his bike. I discovered afterward that neighbours banded together and replaced his bike. He ended up with his heart broken but fixed.

Her death was a peaceful one. Soon after I arrived, family and friends started to gather at the house. The mother was still at home. There were lots of tears, people telling stories and bringing food over.

I find that rural communities tend to home in and support each other. In this community, the neighbours knew that the mother was sick and the father couldn't work. He stayed home to help her and the kids. He became the primary caregiver. Finances were tight, but it all worked out.

Kerry clearly was able to meet the child at his place in time. Words are important, and she uses the right words to connect. It changed the whole meaning of things for this child and how he will remember the event.

Do Not Resuscitate
Helen's Story

I was in my first year of nursing on a cardiac unit at a children's hospital in the mid-1980s. My patient was an infant who was only weeks old, with a severe heart defect. The family had decided they would spare him the numerous painful surgeries that would be required to "fix" his cardiac defect and deemed him a do-not-resuscitate (DNR).

One day, I was giving him his bed bath and had removed his cardiac leads. Shortly after his bath, he became distressed. The physician and our nurse educator happened to be in the room with me, assessing other patients, when I called them over. The physician assessed and agreed the baby was bradycardic [had a slow heartbeat] and confirmed his DNR status.

As the three of us stood there watching him in the incubator, I recalled feeling helpless and sad for the infant, because his parents were not present. The nurse educator did something that was so simple, but that I would never forget—she picked up the infant and held him while he passed. I remember thinking at that moment: *No baby came into this world alone, and they should not leave alone either.* That simple but profound gesture stayed with me.

Many years later, on the same unit, my colleague had a patient who was about eight months old. His parents had just left to grab a much-needed break and a coffee. While they were away, the baby went into respiratory and then cardiac arrest. The physician and other nurses were present, and when his DNR status was confirmed, no further actions were taken. Again, we stood there watching him, and I remembered my previous experience. I picked him up and held him while he passed. And I remember, as I held him, whispering in his ear that his parents loved him.

I think it provided some comfort to his parents that he didn't pass alone.

I share this story often. I believe whether it's holding a baby in your arms or holding someone's hand as they pass, it must be comforting when their loved ones are not present.

A Guiding Moment
Michelle's Story

I graduated and officially became a nurse in 1996, but it wasn't until three years later that I felt the true impact of what it meant to have the privilege of calling yourself an RN.

At that time, I had worked at a children's hospital, on the cardiac floor, for two years. While in my third year working there, I decided to take the plunge and cross-train to be able to work in the cardiac ICU. I was looking after some of the sickest babies and young children from across the country. It is funny how life just evolves until one day, you are literally shaken by an experience and your existence gains a whole new meaning and momentum.

My patient, an eighteen-month-old baby boy, had just rolled out of the operating room (OR) after having open-heart surgery. His surgeon and an OR nurse accompanied him to my care. His parents were not even in the room yet. The plan was to get him comfortable and settled; then I would go and get them and bring them in. I could hardly see him in the crib for all the wires and tubes connected to his peacefully sleeping body. His sternum was still open, with a clear sterile covering, to give the inflammation in his chest cavity time to decrease so in a few days, it could be fully closed. We would keep him completely sedated until that time.

He had not been in the room fifteen minutes when his heart completely stopped, and so did my world. Thankfully, the surgeon was still in the room. A code blue was called, and the surgeon reopened the sterile covering to get at his heart. As he ran to get the internal paddles, he yelled for me to reach in and massage the heart. I think I was in V-tach [a fast, abnormal heart rhythm] myself as I reached in and gently kept this baby alive with my hands.

This only lasted thirty seconds until they were able to use the paddles and restart his heart. Thankfully that was the kick-start he needed, and eventually he recovered.

It was also the kick-start I needed, as I felt the wave of change wash over me. It took four years of nursing school and three years of practical nursing care before I faced the enormous impact of what it meant to be an RN. The circle of life, and the role I can play within it, is a gift that I grabbed hold of that day. I never looked back. Through all the devastation and all the joy, that moment has guided my nursing career ship to this day, some twenty-four years later, and will continue to be my beacon of light.

Working with Children
Sue's Story

For nurses, time, consistency, and familiarity can build relationships. You often see this in nursing homes, long-term dialysis units, rehabilitation units, and other situations.

My story is about a little guy I looked after on the pediatric ward of a hospital. I got into pediatrics quite early in my career. My first job in the early 1970s was in pediatrics. At some point I did geriatrics, and then later ended up back in pediatrics.

The child I'm thinking of grew up on a unit of the hospital. He was born full-term but had a diagnosis of broncho-pulmonary dysplasia. This is a condition in which the lungs don't mature as the child is growing. He had breathing problems and was on oxygen. From day one, he had a lot of challenges. He was the cutest little thing. He was almost two years of age when he passed away. He never did learn to talk. His room was next to the nursing station, and from his crib, he would watch people come and go—passing the nursing station. He became familiar with people and things. One of his favourite things to do was watch television and movies. We would have to disguise the TV if we moved it into another child's room. This was because he would get upset, jump up and down in his crib, and with this excitement he would turn blue. He was de-compensated, and this caused him to turn blue due to his lack of oxygen. We spent a lot of time with him and he captured our hearts. We got very attached to his mom, who visited him regularly. His dad was home looking after the other children. You had to love this boy. He was so full of energy and had a beautiful smile.

I believe he is the reason I stayed working with kids. Adults would get sick and complain, but I found that children would get sick and their main goal was to get well enough to get to the playroom. Children live in the moment and their focus is play. A lot of people would question why I worked with children. Some questioned how it didn't break my heart. I got so much joy working with kids, playing with them, interacting with them. Yes, it does break your heart, but you just can't stop doing it.

MARIAN FACCIOLO

Dying In a Retirement Home
Debbie's Story

In the next story, Debbie talks about her bond with an elderly couple and death. She describes how she was able to influence the outcome and provide comfort through the dying process. Sometimes this is as simple as anticipating and understanding needs.

I was a student nurse studying for my baccalaureate degree and working part-time as a registered practical nurse at a retirement home (RH). I was caring for an elderly gentleman who was well into his nineties. The patient was palliative, with a slow decline. He had stopped eating and had taken to his bed. He had been in his bed for four or five days. All the staff knew that he was palliative—gradually fading away. There was no real underlying significant disease that I can recall. He lived with his elderly wife in the RH. They shared a room and a queen-size bed.

His wife called the nursing station the day I was working. She wanted someone to come and check on him, as he was having difficulty. She was concerned because her husband had stopped taking sips of water. He was semi-conscious, and he had shallow breathing.

I went up to his room. His wife was lying beside him in the bed. He was trying to reach out to her but didn't have the strength, and she was lying there stroking his head and talking to him. She was having trouble maintaining physical contact with him, as she too was elderly and frail. I went into the room and took his blood pressure, pulse, and respirations. I could tell he was slipping away. I asked her if she wanted anyone called, but she said no, they had no children or family.

Initially, I sat at the side of the bed and she told me about his life, how they met, and how their life had evolved. She told me about their love story. I could see he was trying to reach out for her. He was weak, but had purposeful movements. I got into the bed, lay down on the other side of him and helped him roll over so he could face her on his side. I used my body as leverage so he could be on his side and cradle her. We lay there for about twenty minutes to half an hour. Doing this allowed one of his arms to cradle her. We talked about what he meant to her, and she told him how much she loved him.

At some point, it was evident that his respiratory status had changed. He stopped breathing. His spirit was gone. His wife said her goodbyes and was eventually able to let him go. After he passed away, we stayed there for about an hour. We stayed there like that until she started to feel his body cool. Then she was ready to let go.

The doctor was called. The death was pronounced.

Those memories of palliation had an impact on me. Having this experience was a stepping-stone for me. I realized that the dying process, and helping someone have a peaceful and memorable death, made a difference for me. Death was a beautiful and natural process. This experience allowed me to work through my own fear of death. It was part of the reason that I ended up going into palliative care.

Snapshots of Death and Dying
Sharon's Story

I remember I had been out in the workforce but went back to school to study to be a nurse. As a student nurse, I remember feeling afraid of being with that first dead body. I remember, after a death, going in with the staff nurse to prepare the body. I felt nothing at all. I was totally devoid of any feelings. I didn't know the person. I had had no interaction with the person prior to putting a toe tag on his body. My job was to wrap the body. No feelings from me that time. It was very strange.

When I first went to work as a nurse, I ended up working on an oncology unit. I was working the night shift. It was two or three in the morning. We did our rounds. I went into a patient's room and could hear heavy, deep, slow breaths followed by a long period of silence. She was "Cheyne-Stoking." That is what can happen before a person dies. I can hear the sound now as if it was yesterday. Each time I did rounds that night, I could hear that sound. You never forget that sound once you have heard it. I remember she was emaciated. I remember the sound of her breathing. I remember how long it took her to die. The next night she was still there and still Cheyne-stoking. She ended up dying that second night. I had to wrap the body. I kept thinking she would start that deep, slow, abnormal breathing and then stop altogether and then start over. I thought she would resume breathing while I was wrapping her body. I was afraid.

Once, I went into the room of a patient who did not have a do-not-resuscitate (DNR) on his file. I was also on the "code team." This meant if a person died without a DNR in place, we (the code team) were responsible to start resuscitation. We were legally responsible to respect their decision and do a code. Doing resuscitation on palliative patients is very difficult for me. I describe it as if when the person is passing and letting go, you do a big "thump" on their chest. They have taken their last breath and are transitioning to the next life, and you "thump" and disturb their spirit. You are calling them back. It feels like you are disrupting the peaceful and normal process. I believe my feelings are concerned with the quality of life and dignity of dying. With that dignity in death, a nurse wants it to be as peaceful a process as possible for the person. This is why I believe in having a DNR in place when people are dying. It reminds me of Gilda Radner's book *It's Always Something*. I find it so true to oncology and palliative care. I think that working with dying people has made me understand and appreciate the need for advance care planning.

I remember this one man who was on the oncology unit who had leukemia. He was so sick, he couldn't get out of hospital to celebrate his fiftieth anniversary. He had a large family. They brought him a beautiful picture and they came in to celebrate his anniversary. Eventually he did go home, but he came back a couple of months later. He finally died in hospital. I believe we supported him through to his death. We helped the family support him.

This is so different from another man who I cared for on the same unit. He was afraid of dying. He had no one. He too was dying, but he was alone. The night of his death, I spent a lot of time with him. I sat by his bedside, made sure he was clean and comfortable, held his hand, was there with him. There was a code called on another patient that night. I did all I could to spend as much time as possible with him. He had nobody else. It was important for me to be there with him.

As I tell these things, they are fresh in my mind from twenty years ago. Parts of the stories have stayed with me. I think I remember because of the people involved and the people with whom I made the connection. I can see faces but can't remember the names. I remember parts of the stories. I remember the connections that were made. There were some I couldn't connect with at all. I think it is important to get to know the patients you are working with. I think that all my experiences have taught me how to do an excellent assessment. I can pick things up by just looking at the physical signs (edema, cyanosis, breath sounds, etc.). I like to get to know patients, and their families. It helps to know when something is not right.

There was one lady who was a lawyer. She was diagnosed with cancer and spent a lot of time on our unit. She was with us for some time, and we got to know her well. She had a lot of oncology treatment done while on our unit and was so upset about her hair falling out. Although terminal, she would sometimes get day passes to leave the hospital. We would get orders for special things, like an aperitif such as Tia Maria. Imagine having to get an order for a drink for a dying person. This was in the 1980s and in the hospital. Her friends moved her from one house to another. She didn't get a chance to spend much time in her new place. Her friends did a VHS movie of the move. We used to joke with her. I will always remember her.

Sharon acknowledges the importance of the connection with the patients in her care. She remembers people as "snapshots" in time. Notice that she does not refer to the pain medication or other therapeutic interventions, which were important and needed. She does remember the essence of the patients involved and some of her own feelings.

MARIAN FACCIOLO

Dying Oncology Patient
Debbie's Story

I was a third-year nursing student, working in the oncology department, when I met a young woman who had just been diagnosed with lung cancer. She had clubbing of the fingers, and other signs were there to indicate the severity of her condition. The patient had come in for her first chemotherapy treatment, and as a student, I wasn't yet able to start intravenous therapy. I was not doing the other medical tasks that the staff nurses were busy doing. I had the time and opportunity to talk with the patient.

She was in her mid-thirties and had a newborn baby. She told me how she'd had trouble conceiving and had been on hormone therapy for about five years. Finally, she got pregnant. Five or six months into the pregnancy, she started having a persistent cough. She declined quickly. The baby was delivered at about eight months when it was discovered the patient had lung cancer.

She looked me straight in the eye and told me, "I want the truth. I have things to do, and I want my daughter to have a memory of me. They tell me they are going to do this, and they are going to do that. They have this statistic and that statistic, but… I want the truth, and I need the truth. I have things to do."

It was hard to do, but I went to the oncologist and told him what the patient had said to me. He drew the curtain and sat down to speak with her. I could hear her sobbing. After he left, I remember just holding her. She cried and cried. She had only weeks or months, even with treatment.

She knew the truth. She knew in her heart that she was dying. She felt that people were telling her things and giving her false hope. Although she wanted to believe it, she knew it wasn't the truth.

She made a video for her daughter and told her about her own journey and how much she wanted her and how much she loved her. She never did get the chemotherapy, and I never saw her again. I did hear that she died with the baby beside her. The baby was only six weeks old. She wanted to leave her daughter something tangible of her and she managed to do that.

This was my first experience with the community of cancer. There is a community of like-minded disease where they celebrate and mourn together. It was an enlightening experience to be part of this unit.

Trust and Personal Connection
Marian's Story

It was an intense time when I did my student practicum in psychiatry at the Douglas hospital in Montreal. I remember vividly that there were many times when our emotions, either as individuals or as a group, were extremely high. In order to complete the placement, we each had to pack our bags and leave the comfort zone of the nursing residence. We took a bus together to the mental health hospital, where we lived and worked for three months. During that time, we learned about psychiatry and worked on different floors with different populations. It was a journey of exploration, as we learned not only theory but also a lot about each other and ourselves. We formed relationships with many of the patients who also lived in the hospital. Some patients had lived there at the psychiatric unit long-term. Others were expected to be there for assessment, crisis or a short-term stay only.

I was placed on a floor with another student nurse. The people on that ward were young adults to middle-aged, both male and female.

The unit had trained nurses, orderlies, and a psychiatrist. The male psychiatrist had regular group sessions. He invited my classmate and me to join these sessions with him. I remember that it was as if he was the father figure and we were either the mothers or perhaps the sisters. In any case, as a group we sat around in a circle; everyone talked about how their day or week was going and the challenges that they might be facing.

It was on this ward that I met Robert. He was tall, over six feet, with a large frame. He was quite young. I remember he wasn't much older than I was at the time. It made me curious and a bit uncomfortable to be with people so close to my age. I wanted to know what brought them here and how they ended up the way they did. I wondered about what the future held for each one of them. It was expected that we would do the research and read their file so we could get the background on each one. We did what was expected. I was often still puzzled.

Robert was depressed and in his early twenties. He took part in the sessions but never said much. He would just sit there and look around as if uninterested. I do remember that we did talk one-on-one a few times. He was obviously broken, medicated, and bottled up with emotion.

One day, a few hours after one of these sessions, Robert got really agitated and angry. He started to shout and throw things. He picked up a chair, threw it across the room, and it hit the wall. The psychiatrist who worked with Robert wasn't on the ward at the time. He was called to come urgently. It wasn't long after the chair was thrown that the doctor arrived. He must have given a verbal order for sedation, because when he arrived, the nurse had already drawn up the sedation and was ready to give Robert the needle.

This was when I was most frightened. Robert had retreated into his own room; there was havoc everywhere as staff circled Robert in his room. The doctor came into the room and Robert lunged at him. The male orderlies quickly restrained him; the needle was launched, the straitjacket put in place. I was thankful that the staff acted swiftly and were able to protect the psychiatrist and Robert himself. I just stood there and watched. I think I was in shock.

They got Robert onto the stretcher and put the side rails up. He was going to an area where he could be monitored more closely. As they put the rails up and started to take him away, Robert, now restrained, sounded helpless and cried over and over, "I want Marian to come with me… I want Marian to come with me."

I couldn't believe my ears. He wanted me to go with him. I cringed inside. I thought to myself, *Why me?* I was frightened and started to tremble. I didn't know how to react but felt that I was probably safe to walk beside the stretcher. I got a nod from the psychiatrist, who was still there. I walked over to the stretcher as the two orderlies moved it down the hall. The only noise I heard was the sound of my knees knocking together as I accompanied Robert to the observation room on another unit. He didn't cry out anymore. He settled right down. I'm sure the medication was starting to work.

I still, to this day, remember this incident. He wanted me to go with him. I do know that I'm glad I did this and that he viewed me as someone he could trust. I will never forget Robert and that day on the ward with him.

Trust and positive regard are an integral part of the nursing relationships. In this instance, I am not sure why Robert trusted me. Prior to this incident we did have a couple of one-on-one conversations together. As a student, I did not have the same workload or level of responsibility that staff on the unit had. Perhaps this allowed me the time to be fully present. Robert was also closer in age to me than he was to some of the staff providing care at the hospital. I believe all these factors may have played a part. There are also unknown factors that play into why some people connect with certain people more than others.

The Joy of Twins
Mary's Story

While working for a pediatric agency, I was assigned to three-year-old identical twin boys who had been born three months premature. They both had severe spastic cerebral palsy.

In the morning when I arrived, they would hear my voice and squeal. Their little bodies would be very rigid and spastic from not moving all night. Number One twin was slightly less compromised than his brother, who was blind. Neither of them could speak. Both had seizures, difficulty swallowing, breathing issues, incontinence of urine and stool. They wore diapers and ate only pureed foods.

Each morning started with inhalation treatments and the administration of many medications. Next they lay in a warm bath to relax their small, rigid bodies. I would work their bodies, starting with turning their heads gently back and forth, working my way down their bodies until their toes and feet were done. Slowly they loosened up. Doing these tasks took until lunchtime. Feeding them took between an hour and an hour and a half.

After lunch was their favourite time. We had about an hour and a half to go to the park. I used a double stroller. When I mentioned going to the park, they would both let out squeals. At the park, they liked me to put them on the slide and hold them while they went down. Each time, they'd squeal with delight. They also loved the swing.

One day, I was observing Twin One as he watched a little boy sitting at the picnic bench. The little boy was sitting facing outward with his legs swinging. I took Twin One out of the stroller and brought him over to sit beside the little boy. I needed to support him completely as he didn't have the strength in his torso to hold himself up. He squealed and squealed with delight. It was such a little thing, but it brought him so much pleasure. Before too long we tried the teeter-totter. It brought the same squeals of joy.

Of course, I had to explain carefully and without too much information to the little boy and his mom that there was a developmental delay with the twins. I was careful to honour the privacy and confidentiality of the people involved. Often, the same boy and mother would make a point of going to the park to play with the one twin.

The boys usually fell asleep on the way home from the park. At about two in the afternoon, either a physiotherapist or an occupational therapist came to work with the twins. These therapists showed me things to work on with them to improve their function.

I will always remember one day with Twin One. Both boys had special wheelchairs to which I could attach a table. On Twin One's table, I put one red and one blue plastic ring within his reach so he could grab them. Repeatedly,, for weeks I would say "red" when he grabbed the red one and "blue" when he grabbed the blue one. Then one day I said, "Get the red one. Get the blue one." He knew one colour from the other. He squealed and squealed after he got it right. He knew the difference and was proud of himself. That week he learned all the primary colours. It was a special moment for me, but it was an even bigger moment for him.

We did warm water (I said "hot") and cold water, and eventually he learned that as well. Twin One would always make a sound when his hands hit the water. They had different expressions for the different temperatures of the water. They had a hidden brain working inside. I tried rubbing their skin with soft fabric and rough fabric. When I did this, they would get serious. I would tell the boys which one was soft and which was rough, and then rub it on their skin. They loved it. It was like a game to them. They loved music and they would sway and squeal when I played it for them. Ripping paper put Twin Two into a fit of laughter. When I ripped Velcro, it caused them to laugh. I loved to make them laugh. Twin Two was blind, so whenever there was an unexpected sound, he would jump or cry.

I spent three years with these lovely boys. If they caught a cold, it would quickly go to pneumonia. I had to monitor their medical status, as they were very fragile. Sometimes if they had a severe seizure, I would have to call an ambulance and one or both would be admitted to Sick Children's Hospital for a couple of days or maybe even weeks, depending on what was wrong. If one went to hospital and the other stayed home, they made you aware that they missed their brother. They were just not themselves. They were medically fragile boys who spent a lot of time in the hospital. The nurses in the hospital knew them well.

These boys had such a difficult time just staying alive, having so much pain. Watching them with new things or even old pleasures was a joy I will never forget. I understood the joy and can say it is much like the joy a mother feels for her children. I took great pleasure in watching them when they were learning new things and overcoming barriers. I watched them progress and took great pride in their accomplishments and my involvement with their learning.

Twin One was walking with a walker when they moved on to a different care level.

In this story, Mary describes providing shift nursing in the home environment over a relatively long period of time. She provides nursing care and respite for the family. There is consistency and continuity of care, which is related to the need, setting and circumstance. Mary's effectiveness with the twins is related to her medical knowledge, her knowledge of normal growth and development, her strong attachment to the boys, and her commitment to the relationship.

5. Intuition and Experience

Science, art, self-knowledge, and ethics work in concert as ways of knowing in nursing. Another important aspect of nursing is the ability to learn from and build on experience. I later came to realize that there is another vital dimension to effective nursing. This other factor is gut feeling or intuition. Over the course of my career, I have come to rely on and trust my intuition. Throughout this book the value of experience and intuition is highlighted in many of the shared stories.

Experience as a Public Health Nurse
Lois's Story

I was a public health nurse (PHN) in the days when we got referrals from agencies like the Children's Aid Society (CAS). One day, the request was for a nurse to visit and follow up with a young family. The family was being monitored by a PHN, who I was going to replace.

I first met the family on a joint visit with this other PHN. I was a bit intimidated by the father, as I had been told that the man had thrown a

CAS worker down the stairs. This happened when the couple lived in their previous apartment, and it happened with a CAS worker who was involved with them at the time. Obviously, they did not have a good rapport with the worker who was thrown down the stairs.

The PHN who I was with during my initial visit was seeing and following the couple, partly because the father had had this altercation with a CAS worker. This was why there were two of us doing the visit. There were also some concerns about the safety and well-being of the children. The couple had two little girls, ages five and seven. They now lived in a small rented house in the country. Monthly visits were being done to monitor the home situation. During the visit, the PHN I was with had accepted a cup of coffee. She was working on her rapport with them. The couple went to their tiny kitchen and came back with two cups of coffee, one for me and one for the other nurse. There were all kinds of old coffee drips down the outside of the cup. I really didn't want to have the coffee, but I didn't want to offend them either. So I pretended to take sips now and again.

The parents were quite cooperative. Both the mother and father were always there. I carried on with the monthly visits and made these "surprise" visits. I always had to make sure I had another visit in the area in case the family wasn't home. I made these monthly visits over a period of several months. I could tell that the seven-year-old was very needy. While I was speaking with either her mom or her dad, she would sit very close to me and take my ponytail and fiddle with it. She would bring out a comb and want to comb my hair. I didn't really like it, but was trying to work on my rapport with her and the family, so I allowed her to do this. I was only twenty-three at the time.

I interpreted her need to be physically close to me as a sign that she needed more attention. Were the parents giving her the attention that she needed? At the time of my visit, they did not seem remotely interested in her.

One time, the seven-year-old accompanied me to my car when I was leaving the home. Her parents weren't with her. She said to me, "Can I come home with you?" I told her, "No, of course you can't." She said again that she really wanted to come home with me. I told her I couldn't do that. I said this, but... I also had a nagging in my gut that something wasn't quite right. I did not know what it was, though. I didn't have any other experience quite like this to compare it to.

About a month later, the little girl was admitted to the Children's Hospital with severe burns to her chest. Her nightgown had caught on fire. The story from the parents was that she got up on the stove when the elements were on.

When she returned home, I revisited. I saw the scars. The family was transferred back into the care of the CAS after that incident. There was a suspicion that the children had been left unsupervised.

I thought for many years about that little girl and the look on her face when she asked to come home with me. I will never forget that look. It haunts me to this day. I still think of it.

If I had to do it over again, I would do things differently. When the little girl asked to come home with me, I would ask her why she wanted to come home with me. I would not just say, "No, you can't come home with me," and leave. I would explore things. I would ask more questions. Maybe that incident and burn would not have happened to this little girl. I don't know for sure, but I do know I would do things differently.

Here, Lois describes one of her early experiences as a public health nurse. She had graduated a couple of years earlier and did not have a lot of experience. Many years later, she continues to ponder and reflect on the incident. Lois had something nagging at her. Something wasn't right. She felt uneasy. Lois ignored the scratching in her belly. Regardless, it is one more experience to inform her future nursing interventions.

Scenario One: Story of Neglect
Anne's Story

Anne shares a story whereby she talks about her inexperience and anxiety dealing with neglect. As a novice case manager, she is able to build on what she learns in Scenario One so she feels more confident to work out Scenario

Two. With experience, she becomes more attuned to her gut feelings and trusts them. She has moved further on the continuum from novice toward expert nurse in situations related to neglect and abuse. The two stories that Anne recounts illustrate growth in what she knows about herself, others and patients who can be subjects of abuse.

Alice was a seventy-year-old patient suffering from dementia. Our intake department received a call from her younger sister Rose, who was her primary caregiver and lived nearby. Rose informed us that she had met a man online and was going to Vancouver to meet him and would be away for two weeks. As a result, Rose told us that Alice would need some support during those two weeks. The intake case manager was straightforward with the family and explained the referral process and the eligibility criteria. She recommended Rose not leave if the patient needed support in the home and there was nobody to provide that support. She was informed there was a waiting list for personal support workers (PSW) and recommended that Rose make alternative arrangements for her sister's care. Rose was told that an in-home assessment would be done by a community case manager, but that it could be at least a week before the home visit was done, depending on how many new referrals the case manager had to complete.

At the time when this happened, community case managers might have anywhere from 120 to 150 clients on their caseload. We were not considered an emergency service and we didn't provide twenty-four-hour care in the home.

I got the preliminary information and the file was flagged with a request for me to do an urgent home visit. From the initial information, the patient was deemed to need a lot of help, yet Rose was leaving for a vacation. It was the dead of winter and the patient would be left alone. It was made clear that Rose was leaving to meet her new boyfriend.

I booked a joint visit with the PSW supervisor. When we did the visit, Rose had already left.

Alice lived in a very small space. It was an attic apartment. The only access to the apartment was a steep set of external industrial steps. There were approximately fifteen of these steps leading to the entry door. I later confirmed that it was the only entry/exit for the place. As a young, agile person I found it rather dangerous making my way up the slippery steps. Once we made it to the top of the stairs, we found the key to the place was stored on a small ledge over the door. It was not easy for me to retrieve the key, so it would be very difficult and dangerous for Alice. I tensed as I worried what would happen if it fell and landed in the heap of snow below. If the patient dropped the key, how would she find it to gain entry again? She would be left outside in the cold. I held the key tightly and opened the door.

As the door opened, I noticed an unbearable odour of feces and urine. The smell was palpable. I felt my stomach turn. There was no turning back. I had to continue. Once inside, I noticed that a space heater was the only source of heat for the apartment. The local hydro company had been leaving notes stating that work was going to be done and the power would need to be shut off. They didn't give a date for this, only a notice. This patient with dementia would not know how to turn the power back on if it was turned off.

I looked around the apartment and discovered that there was minimal food on the shelves, and whatever was there had expired. There was rotted fruit visible on the counter and an empty fridge. A small dog wandered about the apartment. I determined that the dog was the source of the putrid smell, as it had eliminated on the floor in several locations. The patient was unable to either take care of the dog or take it outside to do its business.

I assessed Alice and determined that her dementia was moderate to severe. She was unable to manage her medications. She should not have been left alone, as she was at risk for falls, especially if she tried to leave her apartment. Although she was walking unaided, she was frail. I could not imagine her navigating the stairs safely. When I asked her how she would manage to take care of herself, she told me that she would walk to the local store to get food. Although it was the middle of winter, she did not seem to be aware of this.

While I was doing the visit, another sister from out of town, who lived a plane ride away, called. I got Alice's permission to speak with her and added her to the contact list. Then I shared my concerns about her sister's safety and well-being. I explained that the authorities might have to become involved. She kept saying to me that she would fly in and help her sister until Rose returned. This never actually happened.

When I returned to the office, I did an urgent follow-up with the management team. I made several attempts to get hold of Rose, to no avail. This was considered an exceptional circumstance, so I received authorization from management to put in twice-a-day visits and night shifts from PSWs to monitor and care for Alice. Out of the goodness of their hearts, the PSWs brought in food and fluids for her. They cared for the dog and cleaned and scrubbed the feces and urine from the floor. They assisted Alice with sponge bathing, ensured she had clean clothing, and they did some housekeeping.

I believe that, as I was a fairly novice nurse, it took a lot out of me to deal with this situation. I felt so anxious and stressed, wondering if this could be happening to this patient. Could this be happening to me? I admit this, but I also believe that many of the steps I took after my visit served to avert a worse situation for this patient.

I believed that Alice was at risk and needed to be in protective care, where her needs could be adequately met. After this short trial at home with our community supports, I called 911. A police wellness visit was then made.

The visiting officer described the apartment as a "tree house." He told me that unless this patient was committed to the hospital by a doctor, their hands were tied. I got a copy of the police report for Alice's agency file/records. I then called Alice's family physician (FP), who provided the needed documentation. A copy of the documentation was faxed to the police, but they said they would only accept the original copy. By the time I knew this, the FP's office was closed.

The paramedics were sent to the home, but by this time, the PSWs had been there for six hours and had cleaned up the apartment. When the paramedics visited, they found the patient to be doing well. According to them, she answered questions appropriately. It is known that patients with dementia can fluctuate in their state of cognition. The paramedics left the home. They did not have the full patient history, nor did they understand the severity of the situation. They did not understand that the patient was high risk and should not be left alone. I spoke with another police officer to request that a second wellness visit be made. I asked that they try to convince the patient to go to hospital. The second police officer did a home visit, but reported there were not any concerns and left the home.

Once again, I called 911, and another paramedic was sent back out to the home. This time I spoke with the paramedic while he was there. He listened to me as I told him about what I had found and why I was concerned. The patient agreed to go to hospital to be checked out and supported. When I knew that Alice was on her way to hospital, I called the emergency geriatric nurse specialist and gave her a full report. She agreed to advocate for the patient to be admitted to hospital until alternative living arrangements could be made and a thorough work-up done. We discussed possible options, such as long-term care (LTC), short-stay respite (SSR), sister flying in, or Rose returning from vacation. It was decided SSR wasn't really an option, as the patient did not meet the requirements of having a set date for a return home. Alice could not afford a retirement home, where she could have had many of her needs met.

Alice was finally admitted to our local hospital on a Friday. I was finally able to sleep, and sleep I did. That same day, I went on a scheduled and much-needed vacation.

While I was gone, another case manager was assigned to Alice's care. Before leaving for vacation, I gave her an update on the situation and all that had happened in a relatively short period of time. I felt that with Alice and the high-risk situation, there needed to be continuity of information and service. It was complicated, and although there was a ton of documentation, I wanted to be sure that another case manager would be able to follow up with things if needed.

When I returned from my two-week vacation, I got an update on what had transpired while I was away. On Monday, three days after she was admitted, Alice was discharged from the hospital to her home. She hadn't been seen by our hospital case manager, a geriatrician or a geriatric nurse specialist. Nothing about her condition changed. I had requested she have a complete work-up done while at the hospital, but this had not happened. Alice was discharged home. The doctor discharged the patient to the care of the cleaning lady who was hired by her sister. The cleaning lady took Alice home and dropped her off there. No one made sure she had food, her prescribed medications, or supervision. She was dropped off and left to fend for herself.

The patient had been home less than twenty-four hours when she wandered over to the local grocery store. She was found there, lost and confused. It was cold and snowing, but she wasn't wearing the appropriate clothing for winter. The owner of the store took Alice back home to her own apartment. Once the covering case manager was informed that the client was home and that she had wandered away, she did an urgent home visit. Do I need to say that Alice was subsequently re-admitted to the hospital? This time, she stayed there until an LTC bed was available.

When Rose returned, the covering case manager had a meeting with her. She advised her of the severity of the situation. She told her that she could potentially be charged by police because she had abandoned her sister. She was informed that the Public Guardian and Trustee would most likely become involved unless she ensured her ongoing safety and had her placed in LTC. Both the LTC facility and the other sister were made aware of the concerns and the need to keep a close eye on the family dynamics to ensure Alice's safety and well-being. Rose agreed to have her placed in LTC.

I learned a lot about being a care case manager through this situation. I learned a lot about myself. I learned that I am prepared to go to great lengths to ensure that my patients are safe from abuse. This was a high-risk situation, and I did what I needed to do. I spent many extra hours following up with people and working on getting Alice the support and protection she needed. Throughout the whole ordeal, I worried constantly about my documentation and nursing license. I had my team and the management behind me. I now understood the lengths to which I would go to take care of my patients and to advocate on their behalf. I had to constantly try to balance my emotions and the stress and come to terms with my own insecurities. I was empowered through this experience and knew that I would bring strength to my next challenge.

I also learned that although there were many professionals in the community, there was often a lack of communication and understanding among us. I found there was a lack of policies that would allow us to proceed with a situation like this that required a multidisciplinary team. I learned to have a strong voice and to believe in myself so I could help others. I just kept pushing. During the whole process, I often doubted myself. I lost a lot of sleep over this. But throughout the ordeal, I knew my gut feeling was right. I also knew I had the supports. My immediate manager was a good support. I had to seek advice or approval at times from other managers, and their advice wasn't always as good or appropriate.

I worked on Friday night to ensure my documentation was in place. I went to the police station to get a copy of their report so it could be added to the client's file. It wasn't available, so I returned on the Monday to get it.

During the weekend, I put in many extra hours to ensure everything was in place and nothing neglected. While dealing with this situation, I also needed to be sure that my other patients had their needs met and follow-up done. I did not get overtime, because our agency didn't generally allow this. The management might say "flex your time," but this was a real challenge, as the workload didn't usually allow for this

Scenario Two: Things Are Not Always as They Seem
Anne's Story

In this story Anne has practical knowledge about the signs of elder abuse and some experience dealing with it. After going through Scenario One, she read more of the literature on the issue in order to enhance her practice.

I was working as a case manager in the community. I got a referral to do a home visit and assessment on Thelma. She was a woman in her mid-seventies. Her spouse, Fred, was around the same age. Their son Ralph lived in the home with them.

Ralph was around forty years old. He had a mild developmental disability and had a dual diagnosis with psychiatric issues. I knew this about their son because he had been receiving services from our agency a year or so earlier. I had been involved with his care. At the time, according to his parents, he had been functioning well independently until one day, he arrived on their doorstep needing their help.

Ralph looked significantly younger than his age. He was short-tempered. I had a gut feeling that there was something not quite right about the family dynamics. At the time, Ralph had physiotherapy treatments but declined personal support. It was determined that he needed medical follow-up. The family physician (FP) made regular home visits. The plan was for Ralph to have follow-up with the FP and a mental health counsellor. He was subsequently discharged from our service, and I went on maternity leave.

I had only been back to work for a couple of months when Ralph called our community agency, asking for help with his mother. The referral came to me, as the family lived in my geographical area. Self/family referral had been in practice for years at our community agency.

I did a home visit and met with Thelma, her husband Fred, and Ralph. From the time of this initial assessment, I found Ralph to be very controlling, overbearing, and manipulative. His hygiene was poor and his thought process flighty. He was quick-tempered with his parents. They remained polite with him. He seemed like another person—not the man I had met before this.

I spoke with all three of them during the interview. Thelma was petite, less than five feet tall. She was well-kept when I first saw her at my assessment visit. She did need to be in a wheelchair, as she couldn't walk on her own. Her affect was flat. Thelma never made eye contact with me throughout the visit.

During the assessment, Fred periodically tried to speak, but Ralph quickly interjected as if to stifle him. He tiptoed around every movement, gesture, or suggestion made by Ralph. His shoulders slumped as if he carried the weight of the world on them. It was obvious to me he was intimidated by his son. He was walking on eggshells.

Ralph said that he had called our agency for help with his mother because he was worried about her. He said his mother recently fell while she was in the bathroom. She could no longer walk and needed to use a wheelchair. His mother's legs were badly bruised. There were a couple of skin tears that had healed over. When I tried to move her leg, Thelma grimaced, but said she didn't have any pain. I advised Thelma, Ralph, and Fred that they needed to follow up with their FP to have tests in order to determine the degree of Thelma's injury. Ralph wasn't keen on getting any more medical tests done or having medical follow-up for his mother.

Ralph did most of the talking throughout the interview. His dad kept looking at me during the visit as if he were trying to tell me something through mental telepathy. He said he was a retired professional. At one point he did say that he felt burned out and that he couldn't do any more. This fact was important, as he was the person who did the cleaning, shopping, banking, snow clearing, and lawncare. He still had his driver's license. The house did look clean and well kept. I didn't look in any of the bedrooms.

I added physiotherapy (PT) for mobilization and an occupational therapist (OT) for a home safety assessment. The family declined the help of a personal support worker. The son said he could manage his mother's personal care. He insisted he could manage and refused any help. He said that he had decided to stay in the same room at night with his mother so his father could get some rest. He said that he now slept in the same room as his mother. There was an ensuite bathroom.

Fred walked me to my car. He took the opportunity to tell me that his son was the root of all their problems. He didn't elaborate except to say that things had changed since he had moved in. He said that he drank too much alcohol and smoked pot and that was a concern to him.

The physiotherapist did do a couple of visits, as did the occupational therapist, but it wasn't long before Ralph declined the services of the therapists, or they would go to the door and there would be no answer. These are called "not seen/not found visits." A couple of times, the PT went to the home only to be told that she couldn't come in. There was always one reason or another for this. The OT was having similar problems. They would set up visits only to have them cancelled at the last minute. As the case manager, I was called to intervene.

Through conversations with the OT and PT, I determined that Ralph was denying his mother professional services and medical attention. The PT wanted Thelma seen by the doctor, but Ralph continued to refuse to have this follow-up done. They also noticed empty alcohol bottles here and there in the home and the smell of marijuana.

I solicited some help with the challenges by requesting the assistance of another case manager who worked with "complex" clients. We decided that a joint home visit would be beneficial. I booked the visit. On our way to the house, I called Ralph (as was routine) to remind him that we were coming. He decided that he did not want us to come. The other case manager and I each had our day planned and had our own cars. We were on route and almost at the home. We spoke briefly and decided to meet a couple of blocks from the house. We parked down the road and called our manager, who was already aware of my concerns. I gave the manager an update and informed her that the son did not want anyone in the home. I wondered if I should call 911 to have the police come and do a wellness check. We decided that my co-worker, the complex case manager, would knock on the door and pretend that she did not know of the visit being cancelled. It isn't my usual way to lie or have any sort of pretense, but I was concerned enough to want to get someone into the home to ensure Thelma was all right. I felt strongly that Thelma needed someone to advocate for her.

My colleague went to the home and spoke with both Ralph and his mother. Thelma seemed to present well. The family agreed to have professional services in the home. There was agreement to have the OT and PT visit. And they finally agreed to have the assistance of a personal support worker in the home to provide personal care for the patient. Ralph was adamant he did not want police involvement. They did not agree that any medical services would be required. When my co-worker informed me that there was agreement, I was surprised. I had serious doubts that Ralph would follow up as planned.

Together, the complex case manager and I managed the care of this client. The complex case manager would be my support person if I needed. She would be the go-to person when I was away. As it turns out, I was scheduled to be off for a few days. I encouraged the complex case manager to keep a close eye on things. I had the feeling that something was very wrong. It was a gut feeling. I didn't have any concrete evidence to prove anything.

The service providers called to book their visits. Once again, Ralph denied them access to assist with his mother's care. The complex case manager insisted that a home visit be made to ensure Thelma's well-being. She told Ralph she would call the authorities if he continued to deny entry.

We did a joint home visit. When we insisted on seeing Thelma, Ralph requested that we give him a few minutes, as he needed to check in on her. He was in his mother's room for more than a few minutes. The other case manager said loudly that she was coming into the room.

Entering the room was like going into a different time zone. It felt like we were entering another planet. Everything was different. The room was a mess. Every corner had articles of clothing or some type of clutter. The stench in the room was of vomit, urine, and stool. There were incontinent pads in the bathroom. Thelma was found lying in bed, soiled up to her neck in urine and stool. The mattress was saturated with urine. Thelma had sanitary pads and incontinent pads taped to her vaginal area. We tried to move her to look at her backside. She cried out loudly in pain with the least bit of movement. My co-worker went to the kitchen and called 911.

Thelma was being held a prisoner in her own home. She was close to death when we found her that day. She was subsequently taken by ambulance and admitted to our local hospital. Thelma was found to have several bedsores—some of them right down to the bone. The son and husband were not allowed to see the patient when she was in hospital. I do know she never returned to her own home.

From my previous elder abuse case and through years as a case manager, I have developed my knowledge and skills. I have more experience now. I am more confident and trust my gut feeling and instincts. My observations are better. I am more acutely aware. I can read between the lines better, watch the body language more, observe behaviours better, and know what they might indicate. I know more what to look for in these situations of abuse. I realize that each abuse case is different. I feel better prepared because I have built on the first experience. I also know the organizational policy and the decision-tree process. I am now on the agency ethics committee and proud to be there. I have something to offer in the way of experience and first-hand knowledge.

Ever since this situation, I can honestly say that I look at patients, families, and situations differently. I find that I look closer, ask more questions, and take in more information about family and support system and the family dynamics. Since then, if ever I question anything and if ever something doesn't seem right, I will make additional home visits. I want to make sure I'm not missing something. I want to make sure that I have the rapport and a presence with the patient and family. I also like to try to get to know my patients without the family being present to influence things.

6. Abuse and Advocacy

We all have our own unique experiences growing up. When my parents became aware that one of their children had been subjected to abuse, they made sure that it would not happen again. Through their actions, I learned that the vulnerable need to be protected. I carried this lesson with me throughout my nursing career. As nurses, each one of us can find ourselves in a position to identify abuse. It can show itself in many forms. It can be in the form of sexual, physical, emotional, and financial abuse. As professionals we have a responsibility to act on the patient's behalf. There are often signs of it. As nurses, with knowledge, experience and a healthy acknowledgment of what information our "gut" provides, we can play an active role to resolve it or mitigate its impact on the victim.

Abuse Calls for Advocacy
Marian's Story

Ruby was a eighty two-year-old lady who had been transferred to our area from a rural area of Ontario. She was transferred from her local hospital to her son's home in our catchment area. This was done to ensure she received the needed support. We would provide community care, and the services were arranged prior to her arrival. Ruby couldn't return to her own home, as she did not have the family support to sustain her there. Her home was also not suitable. It was supposedly very rundown, and there was no running water or heat. She was a long-standing diabetic needing insulin. She had trouble going up or down stairs.

Her son, whom I never met, lived with his wife, Nora. The couple had three adult children who lived out of the province and were not involved. Ruby also had a daughter, Madeline, who was in her early fifties, and a grandson. It was believed that neither of them could manage her care: her grandson wasn't reliable, and her daughter had severe mental health issues.

At the time of my visit, Ruby was struggling with challenges related to mobility, self-care, wound care, and insulin administration. She had diabetic wounds on both her feet. On admission, nursing was involved for insulin administration, family teaching, and wound care. A worker was in place to assist with personal care and do some family relief. Ruby had urine incontinency and needed help with toileting. The occupational therapist was working with Ruby to assess what other equipment would help Ruby function in the new environment. Finances were an issue. However, Ruby did have her old-age pension. A social worker was involved to help the family get financial assistance for equipment and to link Ruby with the Guaranteed Income Supplement. She was not receiving it, but we thought she would likely be eligible as a low-income senior. A physiotherapist worked with Ruby to assess her need for a walker and to improve her strength and mobility.

When I arrived at the home for my initial visit, a large, barking German shepherd ran toward me as I made my way from my car to the house. Terrified, I rushed back to my car, intimidated by his size and ferocity. He was on a rope tied to the front porch. Thankfully, Nora brought him into the house and put him in the basement while I did my visit. This was my first encounter with Ruby and her support person, Nora. Ruby's bedroom was on the main floor of the house. This was good as it meant she did not have to do the stairs. Her daughter, Madeline, had a room in the basement and rarely came upstairs. I didn't meet her until much later.

Nora had a nice smile and seemed concerned for Ruby. She worked at a local care home as a maintenance staff and told me that she intended to do all she could for Ruby. She worked different shifts and was home at changing times. She seemed gentle but troubled. She walked me out to my car, and we stood there talking. I felt there was something not quite right. This was just my gut feeling from the interaction as we stood chatting by my car. Nora seemed to want to talk about private things, but I could feel her holding back. After all, who was I but a stranger to her? I thought she wanted to get something off her chest but just could not do it.

After my initial visit, I called the social worker and gave her a verbal update and added to the care plan. I expressed my concern about Nora, her need to vent, and get more support. She was Ruby's son's partner, and she seemed more involved and concerned than Ruby's son.

A few weeks after my visit, I got a call from the visiting nurse. She called to report that she had serious concerns about the state of Ruby's foot wounds. The nurse was upset and astonished to find that there were maggots in the wound. Ruby's feet were wrapped in bandages. She never wore slippers, so her dressings often got dirty or wet from walking on the floor.

To coordinate the most supportive care plan possible, I organized a conference at the home. All the providers were there, including the family doctor. However, her son did not attend. Nora was there and seemed upset and embarrassed. The family was struggling to provide care for Ruby when our services were not there. Nora was overwhelmed. The providers reported on their progress with Ruby. Everyone talked about the situation, areas of concern, and how things could be improved. As it turned out, the son and some of his friends often spent time in the basement. The providers smelled whiffs of marijuana coming from the basement during some of their visits. They voiced concerns about the home situation and the neglect that became evident over time.

Several weeks passed. Then, on a Friday afternoon, I got a call from the social worker, who had just spoken with Nora. There was a crisis. Ruby's son had assaulted Nora the evening before. The police were called to the home. Nora was afraid for her own well-being and for Ruby and Madeline. The son was very angry and had made threats. Nora feared that he would come home violent. She said that she had seen this side of him on several occasions. She knew him well and believed she had reason to worry.

The social worker was in the process of finding alternative housing for both Ruby and Madeline. She had developed a good rapport with Nora, who trusted her and turned to her for help to escape. Nora confided in the social worker that she felt it was imperative that Ruby be removed from the home. I was asked to stand by, as my help would be needed.

At the end of my workday, I got another call from the social worker. She asked me to join her at the son's home to help them vacate before the son came home. He was expected at six p.m., but she expressed some concern that he might come home earlier than that. She informed me that Nora had found a friend who was willing to have her stay until she could find suitable alternative housing. The social worker worked diligently to find a subsidized room in a retirement home for the patient and her daughter to live. They would share a room there. With teamwork and persistence, we found a solution.

Right after the call, I notified my supervisor of the crisis. She had knowledge and experience of situations of abusive. She was supportive of the plan and agreed that the risks justified our approach. We had to move fast, and we did. We threw their meagre belongings into black garbage bags. Within minutes, we had them both packed and in a taxi on the way to their new home. We followed in our own vehicles. (Agency policy did not allow us to drive patients in our own cars.) We got them settled and I finally got home about eight p.m. I remember feeling exhausted. I also felt very satisfied that I had managed to work so well with the social worker and family member in order to successfully advocate for both my patient and her daughter. That night I slept like a baby.

I will never forget this crisis. The women were removed from an abusive and potentially explosive situation, and I felt a flood of relief.

As it turned out, Nora did have a conscience. What she struggled with was the knowledge that her husband, Ruby's son, was using his mother's money for his own needs. Nora couldn't stand by and watch the financial abuse going on any longer. She didn't want any part of it. She finally found the strength to expose Ruby's son and to leave him.

It was a job well done and a real team effort. Years later, I met up with the social worker again. We had a brief conversation as we remembered Ruby's care situation in detail, even after so many years. The social worker told me that she used this case as an example when she spoke to groups about abuse.

In this story, you can see the importance of advocating for this elderly patient. Not only was there financial abuse, but there was a threat of physical abuse. There were also signs of neglect regarding Ruby's personal care and well-being and added concerns for Madeline and her well-being.

Advocacy in Hemodialysis
Kelly's Story

I have been a registered nurse for twenty-five years. I spent the first twelve years of my nursing career working in dialysis, and I consider my time there a highlight of my career. I often think back to the many patients I have provided care for.

As I think back, one event always comes to mind. It was what I thought was going to be a typical day on a very busy nephrology unit. I had no inkling the events of that day would stay with me and ultimately make me truly understand the lasting impact a nurse can have on a person's life.

Working with dialysis patients often means you care for and get to know your patients and their families well. People who need dialysis over a long period of time come to the dialysis unit for treatment several times a week so the artificial kidney can do the work that the diseased kidney is unable to do to keep the person alive.

Jeff was a dialysis patient who had been coming to our unit for some time. Both he and his family were well-known to me and the other nurses. Not only did Jeff need renal dialysis, but he was also a person with developmental disabilities. I got to know him over the years. He was a very special person and I always looked forward to seeing him. He was fortunate to have a wonderful and very supportive family.

Unfortunately, one weekend while I was working, Jeff became very ill and his mother brought him to the hospital. He was admitted to the nephrology unit. The doctor working that weekend was not his primary nephrologist. The covering physician came into the unit and did his rounds. He saw Jeff and his mother on those rounds. After the doctor left the unit, Jeff's mother confided in me that she felt concerned that the covering nephrologist didn't really know her son and did not understand how ill he was. She told me how she felt about the physician and confided to me that she felt he was marginalizing her son due to his developmental disabilities. I had worked with that physician for a long time and did not agree with her assessment of him. I appreciated the fact that she felt comfortable enough with me to be open and honest and express her thoughts and concerns. She knew her son well and believed he was gravely ill and should be transferred to the ICU for treatment. I listened to her, provided emotional support, and continued to monitor Jeff on the unit.

Later that day, when the doctor made another visit to the unit, I gently took him aside, provided him an update on Jeff's medical condition and made him aware of mom's concerns. A decision was made to transfer Jeff to the ICU where, thankfully, his condition improved. He was eventually discharged home. It was a long time after this event that I came to really understand the impact I'd had on this family.

Years later, I was still working in dialysis when I got married. Jeff's mother gave me a card to congratulate me. Inside that card were not only her well-wishes for my wedding but also a few words of thanks. She mentioned her gratitude for what I had done that day for her and her son. She thanked me for my actions that weekend a long time ago and told me she believed my actions helped save her son's life. She believed my actions were why she still had her son with her.

I carry those thoughts of gratitude with me to this day. Nurses are educated and trained to recognize the needs of their patients and caregivers. Sometimes we don't realize the impact our assessments, skills, and interventions can have on others.

FRONT LINE NURSING STORIES

I Am Part of the Problem
Marian's Story

I was working in hemodialysis. It was in the basement of the hospital. Our unit had a wonderful group of dedicated nurses and a couple of nephrologists. As nurses, we felt valued by the physicians and by the patients who came for dialysis two to three times a week. There was a lot of respect between the doctors, nurses, and patients who came to the unit daily. We had regular conferences where we reviewed each patient's status. We had a nutritionist and social worker who attended the conferences along with the doctors and nurses. I felt we were a real team. I would go further than this and say we were like a family.

The process of doing the dialysis was acute. By this, I mean that the patients needed precise technique in setup, monitoring, and completion of treatment. Being on dialysis required frequent monitoring of blood flow in and out of intravenous lines through machines to patients. Nurses needed to be vigilant throughout the treatment for adverse effects. Some of the side effects included nausea, muscle cramps, and falling blood pressure with potential shock. The patients who came to the unit for regular treatment were chronic in their condition. We got to know them well, and they got to know and trust us as caregivers.

At the beginning of each shift, it was the nurses' job to prime the artificial kidneys and get them ready for the patients coming in for treatment. Once that was done, we proceeded to each patient in order to "needle" them. This was a term used to describe the insertion of the intravenous line (needle) to initiate and maintain the treatment to clean the blood of products that a kidney would normally clear.

On this day, as on other days, each nurse went to different patients to do this task. I went over to Alice to initiate the procedure that would take a few hours to complete. She was one patient who always seemed to be complaining about something. Sometimes it was about having to be needled, often about how sick she felt during the procedure. Prior to this day, I had noticed that a couple of my colleagues were weary of Alice. I believe it was related to her constant complaining.

On this day, I felt some irritability. Preparing the machines and needling can cause some anxiety until all the patients are up and running with the treatment. I started to needle Alice. I don't remember what she said, but her negativity was grating on my nerves. I don't remember what my non-verbal behaviour might have been.

I do recall that my co-worker Pauline was "needling" someone else beside me. We worked in close quarters and there was little privacy. Pauline looked up at me and looked me squarely in the eyes and said, "I guess Alice really has problems now!"

I was taken aback. I had to admit that Pauline was right. This lady had the misfortune of having a chronic illness that required her to sit in a reclining chair for several hours a day, three times a week. She had the misfortune of needing to have her blood drained through intravenous lines, using a pump and machine to clean that blood and return it to her body. She did not need me, beside her, lacking in empathy for her situation. I needed to be supportive and demonstrate that support.

By the end of the treatment, many of these patients are completely washed out and exhausted. A well person who doesn't need dialysis gets the by-products of living cleaned from their blood by healthy kidneys, and this happens continuously, 24/7. I know I would not have liked to be in the place of any one of these patients who needed these extreme measures to live. Although I was not perfect, I had always considered myself empathetic. I considered myself to be a good nurse. On that day, I was not that person. Pauline had the guts to call me out on my lack of support.

When Pauline looked me in the eyes and said what she said to me, I understood what she meant, and she knew that she had gotten her message across. I will always remember this and am grateful for my co-worker calling me on it. I think that the experience helped make me a better person and a better nurse.

FRONT LINE NURSING STORIES

Advocacy for a Couple in the Health Care System
Barbara's Story

I received a new referral. The initial information made it clear that it was going to be a challenging and complex case. At the time, some referrals were identified that way for different reasons. It could be that many community agencies were involved, it was a high-risk situation, or it involved end of life or any number of situations that require certain levels of expertise. It could be a referral with complexity related to the family dynamics and elements of risk.

This referral was for Stella, an eighty-five-year-old woman living alone in the community. She was living alone because her caregiver husband, Jim, had been admitted to the local hospital with a stroke. The referral came to us from Stella's neighbour, Brenda, who asked to be present at the time of the interview and home visit. Brenda, who lived close by, had been staying with Stella for several weeks. She had basically moved in with Stella, going home daily to change her clothes and shower. She had taken Stella to see Jim at the hospital a few times.

Brenda was retired and in her sixties. She was kind and very concerned about Stella's home situation. She was also concerned that since Jim's admission to hospital, she no longer had a life of her own. She couldn't leave Stella for very long. She was not able to go out to church or visit her own family, as Stella required constant supervision.

Prior to this crisis, Jim and Stella had hired Brenda to do their cleaning, laundry, and shopping. She would stay with Stella if Jim needed to go out to the bank or do errands. Most recently, Jim had lost his licence, so Brenda would drive them around to medical and other appointments. The couple paid her to do these things, and this supplemented her pension.

Jim was Stella's caregiver, and he did the cooking. Stella had dementia and it wasn't safe for her to be left alone. She couldn't manage on her own, but surprisingly, she was able to do her own bathing and change her own Depends. She had urine incontinency but still used the bathroom toilet for bowel movements. She kept her private area clean and would let Brenda know when she needed to purchase more Depends. Brenda kept her stocked.

Jim slept on the main floor, in his own bedroom. Stella's bedroom was downstairs on the lower level. The area was well organized and well lit. It was a finished basement that included a sitting room and full bathroom. The couple functioned this way. The basement room was down a long and open flight of stairs, and I wondered how Stella managed to safely manoeuvre herself to the bottom. Somehow, she did.

When I was introduced to Stella, she barely acknowledged me. She was a short, thin, frail looking lady. Her skin was a pasty colour of white and tight against her bones. She certainly didn't have a lot of wrinkles for a woman of her age. Dressed in her nightgown and slippers, Stella sat in her favourite chair in the den on the main floor. Her chair overlooked the back garden, which was surprisingly well kept. The couple had hired someone to do the gardening and lawn care. The view of the backyard was through a six-foot patio door. The garden had grass and some flowers and was partially fenced. Beyond the property, there was an embarkment leading to a gulley and a major busy highway.

For the interview, I sat close to Stella, who gazed out the patio door window. She was hard of hearing and did not engage in conversation. I had many questions, and Brenda was able to fill in the blanks. She knew the couple well. At one point, I got up from my chair and walked a few feet over to the opposite side of the room—the side with the patio door. The door was jammed with a piece of wood so it couldn't be opened from the outside. This is when I noticed that we were sitting in a raised bungalow. There was a ten-foot drop from the patio door to the ground. There was no deck or patio. It was a sheer drop.

Brenda had called our agency to see if she could get some in-home help for Stella, who couldn't be left alone. On the table in the den, I noticed there were several calling cards and information booklets about our services. I was not the first case manager to make a home visit. Other nurses had been out to see the couple at different times.

Brenda explained that the couple always refused outside help. They were determined to stay at home, and they hired private help only for yard care and snow removal. They did not want to go into a nursing home and refused to make applications, even though they were struggling. She told me that she had befriended the couple. They told her they had no children or family. According to Brenda, these seniors were all alone in this world. They had only one distant relative, from whom they were estranged, who lived in London, England. Brenda told me that they had asked her to take on power of attorney (POA) for both their personal care and their property. She agreed. Brenda was worried that Jim would not be able to come home from hospital and care for his wife again. Not only had he had a stroke, but his mind "wasn't as sharp" as it had been before admission. He was quite frail. While he was in the hospital, he had moments of confusion on more than one occasion when I spoke to him on the phone. He needed help to walk and get out of bed. At this point, Jim was still in charge of his wife's care, so I got permission from him to do the home visit and assess his wife at home.

Before Jim had gone into hospital, looking after the couple was part-time work for Brenda. It gave her spending money, and she still had time and energy to visit her friends and family. She was very involved with her church. She wanted to continue her life the way it had been. She had not signed up for this new role, and she was exhausted.

I did a capacity assessment on Stella. She certainly had cognitive impairments, but when I visited, she was able to tell me that Brenda would take care of her at home. After all, Brenda had been doing this for some time. She told me she didn't want to go to a nursing home and that Brenda would help her with meals, cleaning, and shopping. She forgot who would give her medications.

I was very cautious, as I had been taught to err on the side of caution when doing these capacity assessments. All I was assessing was Stella's capacity to make decisions about going into a nursing home. I thought Stella was borderline for capacity and was cognitively impaired. With dementia, peoples' cognition can fluctuate, so I decided that I would retest or have someone else do it at another time. A person's status can change within the same day and within minutes. Because of her answers, I did not believe that I could judge Stella incapable for making decisions around placement that day. And even if she were deemed incapable, there was no way that Jim would allow her to be taken from her home. I gathered this information from Brenda, from my conversation with Jim, and from the case manager at the hospital. Jim was still her caregiver and in charge, even though he remained in hospital.

I called the hospital case manager and explained my concerns about Jim coming home, considering how frail he was and how much supervision and care his frail wife needed. I kept my supervisor informed of the situation, put in some personal support to help Brenda, and requested an occupational therapist to assess Stella's safety, her equipment needs, and her cognitive state. Stella, in my estimation, was at high risk for physical harm. If she opened the patio door, she would be injured in a fall. She might wander off the property if not supervised, and this could result in serious injuries given that there was a major highway directly behind her home. She was unsteady on her feet and might fall down the stairs trying to get to her bedroom in the basement. She could turn the stove on to make herself a cup of tea and then forget to turn it off. She used a walker only sometimes when on the main floor. It depended on the day and her mood and if someone was there to remind her. These were all possible risks for Stella.

I told my supervisor my concerns and had more than one nightmare about Stella accessing the highway. Brenda felt she was in over her head, and she really did not want the responsibility for looking after Stella, even with the relief help I put in. She cared about Jim and Stella, but she also wanted her life back. She felt consumed by the demands on her.

Brenda called me one morning to say there was going to be a meeting at the hospital. They wanted to send Jim home and were going to discuss the situation. Brenda and Stella were both to attend, as well as the hospital staff on the unit, our hospital case manager and the people who look at the stats related to length of stay in hospital. I advised them that I would plan to be there as well.

We met in the conference room. Jim had been on the rehab unit and had improved a bit physically. He was now able to ambulate short distances with the walker. The hospital staff and discharge planner were there. They spoke about Jim and said they felt he was ready to go home.

I explained the home situation. I said that Jim was returning to a home where he had no family support or supervision. Even with formal support, we could not provide twenty-four-hour care. Not only did Jim need help, but so did Stella. He could not be her main caregiver at this time.

The hospital staff still insisted on their plan. I asked them to look at Jim and Stella as a couple and family. They should not see Jim as a person who needed to be discharged home because they needed the bed. I certainly understood the pressures of the hospital needing the bed. I believe that Jim had become a "bed blocker" to them, and they were adamant that Jim was going home.

I left the meeting feeling frustrated that they did not seem to understand the risks if Jim was discharged home. Stella sat there but was in a different world. She was oblivious to what was going on. She didn't speak and didn't appear to understand what was being said.

I had requested that the hospital staff do a capacity assessment on Jim before sending him home. This wasn't done. Jim was discharged home at the end of the week with the maximum amount of service we could give in the home. He had finally agreed to receive in-home help. However, once he got home, Jim often sent the workers away when they came to the door. This meant we were paying for service that wasn't being provided. Initially, the workers went three times a day, but most of the time he sent them away for one reason or another. Brenda continued to provide some support. I worked out a new plan that Jim could agree to have in place, but he would only accept a limited number of personal support hours.

I did another home visit and capacity assessment, and this time there was no doubt that Stella was incapable of making decisions about placement. Applications were made for both Stella and Jim to go to a nursing home. Jim was very irritable each time a visit was made by either the personal support workers or me. He did not like the interviewing, questioning, and planning. He did not like where he was headed. He felt pressured to do the nursing home application and he didn't like it. But he was also unwilling to hire private help or a live-in companion to enable them to live in their own home. They had the money—that was not the issue. He just didn't want the intrusion of others in his home. Once the paperwork for placement was complete, I was relieved.

A couple of weeks after Jim went home from hospital, and one week after the placement paperwork was done, Brenda called me in a panic. She had gone into the home and found Jim unconscious at the foot of his bed. He was sent by ambulance to the hospital. He'd had a massive heart attack.

Within twenty-four hours of his admission, he died. Stella was admitted to a nursing home as a crisis.

The couple had no friends except Brenda and no family. They had each other and they refused to plan for the day when they would no longer be capable of caring for themselves or each other. They wanted to stay in their own home until the end and at all costs. The outcome could have been worse if something had happened to Stella. It was a good thing Brenda got to the home when she did.

7. Nurses Are People Too

As nurses, our focus is on our patients. We aren't supposed to come to work and think of ourselves or what may be happening in our own lives. When we leave home and go to work, we try to put our personal lives aside and focus on our patients and their needs. Our patients come first, but I think we need to acknowledge that nurses are people too. We have families and lives of our own. Our past and present life events can offer a greater understanding of who we are, how we respond to our environments and, ultimately, what internal dynamics allow us to excel in certain situations and hesitate in other situations. Our experiences shape who we are as people and how we perform as nurses.

Reflections on Practicum Rotations
Marian's Story

Psychiatry Rotation

As a student nurse in 1970, I had an unforgettable journey through my psychiatric affiliation and rotation. Student nurses from our hospital did a three-month rotation at the Douglas hospital which was a mental health centre situated in Montreal. We were expected to pack up our belongings from our permanent student residence and move to the residence at the Douglasl.

While there, we were encouraged to engage in introspection to understand ourselves better, to explore our relationship with each other, and to understand how the group functioned. It made for some intense soul-searching. I remember my time there as an emotional roller coaster.

Meanwhile, the political situation in Quebec was at an all-time high state of volatility and explosiveness due to turmoil caused by English–French relationships in the province. The nationalist group Front de Libération du Québec (FLQ) made front-page news regularly. Between 1963 and 1970, the FLQ detonated several bombs in the city, many of them in mailboxes in the wealthier anglophone areas of Montreal, such as Westmount. There was a bombing at the Montreal Stock Exchange in 1969 that injured twenty-seven people and did extensive damage. Other targets included Montreal City Hall and the Royal Canadian Mounted Police station. By 1970, twenty-three members of the FLQ were in prison, including four convicted of murder. The group kidnapped British diplomat James Cross and Quebec's Deputy Premier, Pierre Laporte. Laporte was later found dead in the trunk of a car. The province was in a crisis. Pierre Trudeau, prime minister at the time, invoked the *War Measures Act*, which allowed the military to patrol the streets and put people in jail without cause. The military also imposed a curfew: people were forbidden to be out on the streets after ten p.m.

I was at the psychiatric hospital when the *War Measures Act* was in place. I don't remember having much contact with the broader community. All my time was spent on the grounds of the hospital and in the buildings there. I don't remember once going beyond this boundary. I was young and not up on the everyday politics except in the broadest terms. I did know that a lot was happening. I had a great sense of fear and apprehension but once the *Act* was in place, I felt safer. After all, I was one of those "maudit anglais" (damned English), as were most of my fellow nursing students. Although my student work at the hospital was not particularly affected at the time, I came to realize that the social and political upheaval had a much bigger impact on my life, my family's life and, consequently, my relationships with my patients, especially francophone ones. There was a high-level sense of "French vs. English" which filtered into the hospital and created tension.

FRONT LINE NURSING STORIES

As nursing students, we got to tour several of the wards at the hospital. One of these was the locked ward for the criminally insane. Although this tour was short, it will forever be imprinted in my mind. Our small group was walked around a large room filled with adult male patients of all ages. We had guards who took us around to make sure that no harm came to us. The tour was very uncomfortable. Some men sat silent, looking dazed; others paced back and forth; some walked around with no particular purpose—either too fast or too slow; and others were having conversations with themselves.

The man I can't forget was sitting on the floor on one side of the room. He appeared to be middle-aged, and he had a very strange look on his face. I was petrified. His eyes were vacant. He sat cross-legged on the floor and dangled a string with something small but heavy on the end of it. He dangled it up and down, over and over, into a hole in the floorboard. Our group stood a few feet from where he was doing this. It struck me as a very odd behaviour. I felt an eerie sense of danger and foreboding as he focused his entire attention on this repetitive action. He was oblivious to our presence.

At that moment, I decided that I did not want to work in mental health as a specialty—in particular, I did not want to work with the criminally insane population. I recognized this was unknown territory for me that I did not want to discover further. I knew that while working with other people I would encounter co-morbidities, including mental health issues. This to me was different from what I observed on the chronic wards of this psychiatric institute.

One expectation during our affiliation was that we would observe electroconvulsive therapy (ECT). I observed treatment of a middle-aged woman. As she lay on a table with limbs restrained and mouthpiece in place, she was administered a jolt of electricity that served to shake her entire body in an intense spasm that almost lifted her from the bed. I thought ECT was inhumane but also acknowledged that I didn't know what the consequences would be if this person were not treated. I vowed that I would do all I could to prevent myself from slipping into an abyss that would necessitate such a drastic measure. I know that mental health conditions and deterioration are complicated. They are not necessarily within a person's control. But during and after those moments of the shock treatment observation, I willed myself to control that which I could in order to avoid not only ECT but also being institutionalized in a mental health centre. I was afraid of what I was seeing.

(I should note that ECT has improved dramatically since those early days, but its use remains controversial.)

Pediatric Rotation While Dealing with Personal Tragedy

In 1971, I was a second-year nursing student doing my affiliation at the Montreal Children's Hospital. At the time, I thought that three months working in pediatrics would be interesting. It never occurred to me that I might like working with kids. In retrospect, after many years working in nursing, this time period presented some of the highs and lows of my career in nursing. It was during this rotation that my family experienced tragedy.

While I lived in residence in Montreal, my parents continued to live in the small rural community on the South Shore of Montreal. My father worked as a policeman for the city of Montreal. Both my parents were fluent in French. There were many English families in the area where they lived, although it was mostly French.

My stint at the children's hospital took place during the FLQ crisis, when Quebec nationalists used terrorist tactics to promote the province's separation from Canada. My dad was a staunch federalist and, as a policeman, he often had to deal with violent pro-separatist activities. One day, on the front page of the newspaper, there was a picture of my dad apprehending a prominent FLQ terrorist. He had the guy in a headlock. This photo presented some peril, not only for my dad, but also for our entire family. I was told much later that the picture and newspaper article led to threatening phone calls to my parents at home. One caller said, "We know who you are, where you live… and we are going to kill you and your family. We plan to get every one of you."

Because of the perceived danger to the family, my parents decided to look for property in Hawkesbury, a community in Ontario close to the Quebec border. My father felt it was close enough for him to commute to his job and still provide some safety for our family.

One weekend, my dad took my mom and the four youngest children to search out some properties there. Apparently, the drive was uneventful, but when he got to Hawkesbury, my dad made a left turn off the main highway. Their car was T-boned by another vehicle. No one died, but my mother went through the windshield. She lay unconscious on the road.

My mother ended up in the ICU, diagnosed with a severe traumatic brain injury. Everyone in the car was injured in the crash in one way or another. My dad had broken ribs. One sister's jaw and nose were broken, requiring immediate surgery. The youngest, who was five at the time, had a minor scalp wound. One brother had kidney trauma and the other was reportedly in shock.

While my mother was in the hospital, she didn't recognize any of us. It must have been very upsetting when her youngest child was allowed to see her for the first time after the accident. My mother looked at her and said, "Who are you?"

For many years. our family referred to this as "the accident." Henceforth, our lives were framed as "before the accident" and "after the accident." It changed all our lives. This catastrophic event resulted in our living with a mom with a severe brain injury. She had changed dramatically.

The accident happened in the 1970s, when a patient with a brain injury was sent home from the hospital without education or support. There was little to no information about the injury itself, what we could expect, or strategies we could use to deal with it all. There was no physical or cognitive rehabilitation or goals for improvement. My mother was sent home with no in-home services or follow-up. Roles changed and relationships changed. We were left to flounder and deal with it on our own. In a real sense, we lost our mother in the accident. I told myself that I was happy that she lived, but I grieved the loss of the person she was before the accident.

I was doing my rotation at Montreal's Children's Hospital when the accident happened. I was told that my fellow nursing students were also informed and had gathered in the common room of the residence to pray for my family. At the time, they didn't know if my mom would live or die. I believe their prayers worked, as she did pull through.

During this time, I decided to immerse myself in my work, devoting my time and energy to the children under my care. In retrospect, I realize this was my way of dealing with the family tragedy. I did visit my mom regularly, although she often didn't recognize me. My father and my older siblings were there to provide her with support.

One of the children I nursed was a young boy around five who was diagnosed with a Wilms' tumour, a kidney tumour that can be fatal if it metastasizes. I cared for this little guy before and after his surgery. I was there, along with his family. I made sure his medical needs were met and that he got all the emotional support I could give. After the surgery, I was told that the tumour was encapsulated, which meant that it was confined. I still like to believe that they were able to remove it without it breaking. The surgeon was very optimistic that they got it all.

Another child was a two-and-a-half-year-old boy with severe eczema. The situation was so severe that he needed to be in isolation. This meant wearing gowns, gloves, and masks to provide care. I had to bathe him and put medicated cream on his skin. Dressings were applied to a couple of areas that were especially bad. These were open, draining, and infected. I needed to make sure he got nourishment in the form of food and fluids and ensure his vital signs and intake/output were good. One thing I will never forget is that he had no visitors. I often wondered where the family was and if they ever came to visit him. It was hard for him to be alone in that crib and in isolation. He would cry or whimper and would scratch his skin. His body, including his face, was scaly, irritated, and red in patches. He seemed to love having someone in the room with him. Once he was bathed and his morning care was complete, I would take him in my arms and rock him in the rocking chair by his crib. He would cry initially; then, with the rocking, he would settle. I could feel his heart beating near mine. As I held him close and rocked, he would eventually become like a "wet rag." He would relax, snuggle in close to me and fall asleep. The closeness seemed to provide the comfort that he needed. I am convinced that this rocking was as much a part of his treatment and healing as the medication, dressings, and isolation technique. I will never forget him and the meaning of those critical times, both for him and for me. I think we helped each other heal. He needed human contact to heal, and I needed him to help me cope with my own recent trauma.

When my rotation was over, exams done and the practicum completed, I was called to speak with Sister Mary Felicitas, the director of nursing. Timidly, I knocked on her door. She called from behind her desk and invited me to enter her office. She eyed me up and down with a very serious expression. Gently, she asked me to take a seat on the other side of her desk. I felt nervous. She had brought me in to tell me that in all the years she had been running the school, mine was one of the best children's evaluations she had ever seen. I did not ask her to explain but knew in my heart the practicum had given me more than I could ever ask for. During that very challenging time, I think dedication to my work carried me through personal pain and crisis to triumph over my own misery. I am very grateful for my time spent working with those kids.

From Hospital to Rehab to Community
Marian's Story

At the time of the next story, I was working in the community as a case manager with complex patients. After working in different areas of nursing for many years, I had a fair amount of both hospital and community experience. The model set up at our agency included people with many different diagnoses. Patients were designated "complex" because of either their diagnosis, a complicated home situation, higher needs, or more risks associated with the situation. Patients with acquired brain injuries (ABI) were included in the complex group. I had worked with ABI patients before, but this patient and family have remained vivid in my memory.

David was assigned to my case load when the referral was made to our agency. My first visit with him and his family was memorable. David was in his twenties. He was short in stature but very muscular, with curly red hair and blue eyes. He was referred to our agency from a rehab unit that had worked with him for some time. David was on the rehab unit after spending many weeks in the ICU, where he had been intubated and connected to life support. David and his girlfriend had been involved in a serious motorcycle accident while driving on a major highway. She died at the crash site, and he ended up with a serious ABI. His life would never be the same. The couple had just graduated from university and they were looking forward to the start of their careers.

Yes, we could work with him and provide in-home rehab and ongoing support, but he would never be the person his parents knew and loved before. They would love this new David, but he would be forever confined to a wheelchair, cognitively impaired, and unable to have an independent life of his own. David's parents were very hopeful that day of admission to our agency. Their goal was to see him walk on his own and live independently.

As a survivor of a parent with a brain injury, it wasn't always easy for me to deal with ABI patients and put my own emotions aside. On the other hand, I had first-hand knowledge and experience of what an ABI entailed and how it could so adversely affect not only the person with the brain injury, but also the entire family. My past personal experience affected me to the core. Sure, it might have happened many years earlier, but such a catastrophic event leaves its scars and imprint forever. The survivors are never really the same. The memory of it resurfaces and the pain continues to be real. As it was in my own family, this family now had two time zones: "before the accident" and "after the accident." At times it was difficult for me to navigate through this as I had three sons of my own around the same age as David. As nurses, we often look at what is happening with our patients and reflect on our own lives and situations. I believe it is normal to do that.

I did the assessment, and it became clear that there was a lot of stress on the parents as they supported him. People with traumatic brain injuries tend to have multiple needs including the management of the impact of the ABI which may include dealing with any emerging behavioural issues. After my assessment, I put David's name on the waiting list for physiotherapy, occupational therapy, social work, and a personal support worker. Waiting lists are a reality in our health care system and can deleteriously affect the healing process. Within the year, one by one the various therapists became involved with David.

People with traumatic brain injuries sometimes develop inappropriate behaviours. It depends on what part of the brain is damaged and the seriousness of it. Some examples of potential behaviours include lack of social judgment, increased impulsivity, inappropriate sexual comments, angry outbursts, acting out physically with bursts of aggression. These characteristics and behaviours are not part of who the person was before the brain damage. They can't control themselves because of the damage to the brain.

David's communication was inappropriate. The behaviour that he exhibited was around sexual comments and innuendoes. This included comments to the care workers, strangers, and me. I could handle it. I had experience with other ABI patients with this and a variety of different behaviours. David's behaviour was evident early. I believe that when this happened his parents were embarrassed. To their credit, they were successful in redirecting him and bringing him back on track. To help manage his inappropriate behaviours a behaviour specialist became involved.

Whenever I did reassessment visits, I included David. However, these visits with him and his parents were lengthy. A visit that would normally take an hour and a half to two hours to complete would take over three hours. David always wanted to give his input. He would perseverate and interject. His mom would frequently remind people that David felt disrespected if you didn't give him your full and undivided attention. It was difficult for him to stay on topic and get his point across. As a result, when I had a conference with the many service providers involved with David's care he was not included. His parents were both strong advocates for their son and brought forth any issues of concern to the meetings.

Working with David and his family was a team effort and required collaboration. It included the family and the team working together. A situation is as simple or complex as the people involved and the family structure that they live and function in. The amount of time it took to do David's care was a consideration for the providers and the management team, who had to address caseload intensity, funding, and resource management.

David's inappropriate behaviours made it difficult to take him on outings as he would often embarrass himself and his parents. When they did go out, his behaviours caused anxiety and at times arguments. On one occasion their intervention was unsuccessful. They were unable to get his behaviour under control. He continued to act out and make inappropriate sexual comments to a member of the public. A big argument ensued. David and his parents had argued before, but these disputes were about things like use of the computer, food, and agreed-on times for activities of daily living. Mom told me this was the worst it had ever gotten. Both dad and mom were in tears! Life with their son was difficult and was taking its toll on them.

It became clear that the parents needed more respite from their caregiving role. They were at high risk for burnout. They came to realize that regularly scheduled respite was necessary if they were going to be able to provide him ongoing support. To ensure that respite was a positive experience for David, staff in the respite home were trained by the behaviour specialist on how to deal effectively with David's inappropriate behaviours.

I worked with several ABI patients over the years. David will always stand out in my mind. It was a challenge to work with him and his family. This is most likely due to his age, the severity of his condition, and the way his accident adversely affected family members and the patient himself. Hopes and dreams were dashed, and it took time, effort, and a lot of fortitude for the family to get through this. I was a mother of sons not far off in age. I witnessed pain, heartbreak, the steady falling apart of the people close to him, and role changes while this family fought to survive and rebuild their lives. I remembered my own past as they struggled to overcome their challenges.

Home at Last
Marian's Story

My mother was living in a nursing home in Quebec. She had a history of traumatic brain injury, though with this initial diagnosis she was physically able to get around and do things. She lived at home until she suffered a massive stroke, which left her unable to ambulate, transfer, or do any self-care. Her speech was not affected, but her dementia was worse. In the hospital, once the acute phase of the stroke was over, they tried to rehabilitate her to get her walking again and at a higher level of function. They were having difficulty, and when there was no progress, they asked us to attend a family meeting at the hospital. After the medical staff heard about the history of brain trauma, they stopped any attempts to improve her physical function. Hence, she was unable to return home. She needed a high level of care. My mother ended up being moved to a nursing home not far from her home. There were family members in and around that area who could visit and provide some support. My husband and I lived in Ontario, so we were limited in how often we were able to visit. She lived in the nursing home for several years.

FRONT LINE NURSING STORIES

In the fall of 2004, my husband and I were planning a trip to Asia in the spring of 2005. One of our sons was teaching English as a second language in Taiwan. We thought it would be wonderful to visit with him there. Both my husband and I had heard exciting things about Thailand. Wouldn't it be nice to make a combined trip to visit our son in Taiwan and then visit Thailand? Thailand was on my bucket list. Our youngest son, who was twelve years old at the time, was still living with us, so we decided we would make the trip over the March break, when he had some time off school. He still would have to be away from school for about three weeks, but we agreed that this was doable. He certainly did not object. We thought he would love it, and besides, it would be very educational. The three of us would go to Taiwan, and our other son who was already there would join us on our trip to Thailand. What an adventure this would be!

Then a tsunami hit Thailand the day after Christmas 2004. There was massive devastation to Thailand and other places, so we cancelled our vacation. My husband was waiting to see how things were in a few months, as he still wanted to make the trip if possible, but there was no way I wanted to venture out there with our younger son. Early in 2005, our furnace broke down. That sealed it for me, as one can't live without a furnace in the middle of winter, and it is a costly piece of equipment to replace. Instead of going to Thailand and Taiwan, we would get the new furnace and visit my mother over the March break. We lived an hour north of Toronto, and the nursing home was about an hour from Montreal, so we had to allow at least eight hours, each way, to make the trip.

Our usual habit was to leave home in the afternoon and reach my sister-in-law's place in Quebec in the evening. We would stay there for the night and venture out to the nursing home in the morning. This time, for some unknown reason, we did it differently. We set out in the early morning, went straight to the nursing home, and arrived there in the late afternoon.

When we walked in, my mother was sitting in her wheelchair in the lobby. I still remember her pale white skin, white hair, and beautiful blue eyes. I called out, "Mommy, it is Marian and Vito." She looked up at us and her whole face changed. She had been sitting there in her wheelchair with a vacant look on her face. When she saw and recognized us, her face beamed with absolute joy. It had been a long time since I had seen her that happy.

Although she did not know we were coming to visit, it seemed as if she had been sitting in the lobby, waiting patiently for us to arrive.

We stayed with my mother for a couple of hours, long enough to help her with her dinner. We couldn't really carry on a conversation because of her cognitive status. She had dementia, which was intensified by her stroke and her past brain trauma. Mostly, we talked and she listened. She enjoyed our company and we were happy to see how much she loved our visit. She always loved my husband, as did my dad. My mother loved his cooking, his sense of humour, and his hugs and affectionate ways. We stayed a bit after dinner, then left to go to the West Island, which we were to call home base for a week.

Not long after dinner, it must have been around eight or nine p.m., we got a call from my brother. My mom had suddenly passed away. She'd had a heart attack. We were in shock! Although she had been unwell and in a nursing home, you are never fully prepared for such things. When you lose your parents, it can feel like you are suddenly an orphan. I had lived with the grief and the loss of the person she was before the accident but now she was gone forever. It was a very sad time.

We stayed in Quebec. My brother made funeral arrangements. My husband was asked to give the eulogy, so we went out to buy him a jacket, dress shirt, and tie.

When I reflect on my mother's unexpected death, I think of how it seemed as if it was all meant to be. We cancelled a family trip to Thailand and instead went to visit my mother. Fortuitously we changed our visit routine. I wondered if this was divine intervention.

I remember some of my palliative patients who died and the timing of their deaths. Many of them were very deteriorated and frail, but they held on for dear life, either unwilling or unable to leave this earth for whatever reason. There were some who seemed to be waiting for permission to leave.

Of course, death is inevitable, but I wonder if people sometimes have the willpower to delay death until some desired event occurs. Did my mother hold on until she was able to say goodbye to me and my husband? At the time of our visit, my mother was not considered palliative. Is it possible that somehow, she decided to let go after we left her? I cared for dying patients who seemed to not want to die until a loved one gave them permission, and they then seemed to depart peacefully.

Long-Standing Abuse
Sharon M.'s Story

This retired nurse talks about her childhood. She has been able to turn a series of challenges into a strength that she shares with other victims of abuse.

I was born in the early 1950s and grew up in a very dysfunctional family. My father was a functioning alcoholic. His priority was himself and buying beers at the neighbourhood tavern for his "friends." My mother was emotionally, physically, and sexually abused by my father. My mother remained in the situation until I was in my teens.

I remember one night when my father was going out drinking and we had no food again. My mother begged my father to leave her some money so she could feed us and pay the rent. This was a time when "children were seen but not heard."

Suddenly, I chastised my mother, blurting out, "Don't beg him. He's not worth it; he's a drunk."

Next thing I knew, I was being choked. I was up against the wall and my father was choking me. I don't remember what happened afterward. I was told that I passed out. After that, I was thrown down the hall of our apartment and my head was hit hard. Apparently after that, my father simply walked out. I presume he went to the bar to have a good time with his "buddies." My mother was quite concerned about me and called her good friend, Mrs. C. Not only was she a good friend, she was also a nurse. When called, she rushed over to our place to check on me. She made sure I was going to be all right. I will always be so grateful to her.

It took a long time for us to get out of this situation. Being young and naïve, my friends would say confidently, "If a man ever laid a hand on me, I would leave," or, "If I ever got pregnant, I would never have an abortion." I always thought this was easier said than done, especially if you are not the one involved in the turmoil. At some point, those same friends did have to make a choice. Interestingly, they stayed in the abusive marriage or did have the abortion.

I understood the reality that it is not easy for a woman to stay. It is not easy to go either. There is fear for herself and her children. If she is uneducated and lacks skills, she might be very fearful about how she might not be able to provide for her children.

Growing up in this environment, working with abuse within a family played a huge part in my nursing career. I carried those memories with me through the three emergency departments that I worked in over the next thirty-five years. They have served me well. I see things from my perspective and understand women who are in abusive relationships. I can defend them and see how courageous these women truly are. When women decide to leave, this is when they are most likely to die at the hands of their partners.

Sexual Abuse and Nursing Experience
Sharon M.'s Story

As a child, I had been sexually abused by two different family members. When the Sexual Assault Care Team (SACT) at my workplace was being set up, I had my RN but was in the process of working toward my BScN. I was assigned to work on the SACT. As the team was being formed, my nightmares bubbled up. The way everything happened, it felt like I was meant to be on this team.

Being part of this team offered me insight into the sexual abuse of kids. Working with the kids afforded me a place to make a difference. I could honestly say to these kids, "It wasn't your fault." While on that team, I was subpoenaed a number of times to court. I became an expert witness. Unfortunately, the SACT was disbanded in favour of social workers. While working with this team, I learned so much about myself.

I am now retired. I must admit that I do miss being a pediatric emergency nurse. I miss acting goofy. The kids gave me permission to do that. The kids gave me so much insight into myself and into kids generally. My years of experience in that area provided a wealth of understanding and, I believe, effectiveness when I transferred to the Poison Centre. When working in the Poison Centre, I got calls from parents and the emergency department staff. I could give the emergency room nurse answers quickly. I could make recommendations. I knew what staff needed to know. For example, they needed to know "Is this patient likely to die or not?" We could then take it from there.

Other times, parents, usually the mom, would call saying "my child," and I would briefly interrupt and say, "Do you mean your two- to three-year-old son?" They would often be amazed and wonder if I had ESP. It really was thanks to my years of experience in the various emergency departments. It offered me that insight. Ages two to three is a very busy and curious age, especially for boys, who tend to be a bit more mischievous.

I Am a Mother Now
Dayle's Story

I graduated from nursing in 2004. I worked in the emergency department of a small rural area of Ontario. We had fourteen acute care beds, three stretcher beds, and two trauma rooms. It was one of my first shifts working there after graduating as a registered nurse.

A young man came in with his two-year-old son. The boy was screaming and crying uncontrollably. He was screaming in pain and for his mother. The boy had been sitting up on the side of his dad's parked truck while his dad stood beside him outside. The young boy fell out of the truck. His forehead hit the ground. When he got to the emergency department, his forehead was bulging. He was screaming and calling repeatedly for his mother. He continued to scream repeatedly. The dad was obviously distressed.

I started to cry. It was not an uncontrollable sobbing but outright crying. I believe the dad saw me. He did not say anything. He was so wrapped up in the emotion of his son. I was there to do the initial assessment of the boy.

As a nurse, you hate to see kids hurt under any circumstance. When you become a mother, it makes it worse. If this had been the same scenario a year earlier, before I'd had my own child, who was now a year old, it would have been different. I remember the tears and trying so hard to swallow and get rid of that lump in my throat.

I will always remember this incident as I know it would have been different if I had not had a child of my own. Now, as a mother of two and being a nurse, there is a different perspective. Your life experience changes, and the roles are expanded. There is an overlap in everything you do as a nurse.

Sick Baby and Mother
Mary's Story

I was seven-and-a-half months pregnant. One of my patients was a lady who had just delivered a baby girl. I did perineal care, helped her get the baby latched on the breast, and changed the baby's diaper. In those days, we did not wear disposable gloves for these tasks. We just washed our hands before and after doing them.

On the third day after birth, the baby was quite lethargic and would not latch on. The mother appeared the same. She was also having cardiac issues. There was enough concern about mother and baby that she was transferred to a Toronto hospital from our general care hospital. I went by ambulance with them. Once they were settled at Women's College, I gave my report and returned to my original hospital.

When I got back to the floor, the other nurses were all in a flap. Apparently, Women's College Hospital had called our unit to inform me that the mother had cytomegalovirus (CMV).

CMV is a common virus, and once a person is infected with it, they retain it for life. Most people don't even know they have it, as it rarely causes problems in healthy people. It usually goes away on its own. It is a cause for concern for people with weakened immune systems or when people are pregnant. There can be severe consequences for babies born with it. These include brain, liver, spleen, lung, and growth problems. The symptoms vary, and there are several. The virus is spread by direct contact with blood, urine, saliva, semen, breast milk, and vaginal fluids. Infants born to mothers infected with CMV can develop the infection. Babies who are infected with CMV before birth are at high risk of several defects, such as small head size, enlarged liver, anemia, pneumonia, vision and hearing loss, and more.

The Toronto hospital reporting back said that a pregnant nurse should not be caring for a woman with this disease. It could be passed along to the pregnant nurse via body secretions and then to the nurse's fetus. They said that there was a chance the baby would be born blind and/or mentally challenged, and so would any other baby this nurse might have.

When I learned this from the other nurses, my heart started to race. I immediately paged my obstetrician, who was downstairs in the auditorium attending a lecture. I called my husband to come to the hospital, and I rushed down to the lecture hall and got my doctor. After telling him what happened, he had blood tests done on me that night and sent them to Toronto.

My hubby and I had to wait three long weeks until the blood results came back. They were negative. We had a healthy baby girl that November.

Nurses have been, and will continue to be, at risk while working with patients, no matter what the setting. Precautions are taken whenever possible. When the medical staff know what they are dealing with, there can be more control. There are many risks associated with blood and body fluids, and universal precautions are used. Nurses are at risk of needle pricks. There are risks associated with blood from others that can ultimately harm nurses as well—for example, hepatitis B, hepatitis C, and HIV. There are many risks associated with respiratory illnesses, too—for example, H1N1, SARS,

MERS and now COVID-19, to name a few. In Mary's case, the scare was that much worse as she had to worry about the possible deleterious effect on her unborn baby.

Death in the Emergency Department
Darlene's Story

I was working in the emergency department and an elderly lady came in by ambulance. She had shortness of breath and gross edema of her extremities. Her difficulty breathing and swollen limbs were signs that she was in end-stage congestive heart failure. Her breathing was very laboured, and her death was imminent. Her medical history and records were pulled so they could be reviewed. The emergency room doctor was an Indo-Canadian man in his early thirties.

I was in the room across from her, drawing up intramuscular morphine for another patient. The doctor came over to me, pulled me aside, and said he needed the medication for this dying lady. He said he needed to keep her comfortable and took the medication from me. He said this lady needed it right away, and he proceeded to give it to her. He asked me to administer oxygen, start an intravenous, and stay with her.

He left the room and returned with the lady's daughter and her two young children. The children were about nine and twelve years of age. The daughter had already spoken with the doctor and understood the gravity of the situation. Then this doctor literally grabbed the children by their shirt collars and brought them to their grandmother's side. He brought them close to her. He held them by the back of their shirts, pushing them toward her.

He said, "Your grandmother is dying." He said, "This is beautiful, and you need to tell her you love her and give her a kiss." He told them this was the nicest thing they could do for her. He was very gentle and soothing. He told them to talk to her, rub her legs, and be with her.

They were on the bed with her when she passed away. She knew they were there, although she didn't talk to them. They did kiss her and rub her but didn't say much at all. They looked stunned and were feeding off the doctor's energy.

What could have been ugly and traumatic turned out to be peaceful, although stressful. He coached them from the side. I watched and I cried and cried. The clergy talked with them, and palliative care was involved.

Later, I told the doctor that I thought what happened was terrible. He looked surprised and said to me, "Why would you say that? It doesn't get any better than that. The kids were with her to comfort her. The family was together, and she died with them around her."

I hadn't expected this from the doctor. I was upset because at the time I was young and understood death in a different way. It was at a time that I was moving myself through the understanding of the dying process. I didn't expect things to go the way they did that day. He was confident in what he was doing. He took charge of things.

In retrospect, I think that he understood dying better than I did. I do know he was from a large family and his roots were from India, but he had grown up in Canada. It was a stressful situation, but he had a calming effect on them. He spoke with certainty and assurance. They listened.

In her story, Darlene presents the dichotomy of her feelings and reactions compared to those of the physician. On reflection, she acknowledges her own struggle with death, dying and what it means to her. She recognizes that we are all individuals and in different states of being and understanding. As a nurse she is also aware that she needs to be cognizant of culture and how this can relate to and effect a person's behaviour. She mentions culture as a variable included both in her analysis initially and with reflection of the situation.

8. Lessons Learned

Part of nursing education includes learning how to analyze situations that have occurred in order to determine the effectiveness of the treatment strategies that were used and to identify gaps so more effective service can be provided in the future. The following stories speak to lessons learned from actual nursing experiences that served to arm the nurse for similar situations and suggest more effective strategies for treatment. The experiences evoked a variety of feelings including happiness, fear and sadness. They provided some valuable lessons.

In the Hospital

He Was Wearing Only a Johnny Shirt
Marian's Story

While telling this story, it needs to be clear that the dignity of the person is paramount. The stories are real-life events, and the patients involved require respect. Sometimes (as in this case), it is the nurse as well as the patient who may be struggling with something new, alien, or even shocking. Patient dignity prevails.

FRONT LINE NURSING STORIES

When I was studying to be a nurse, I was a teenager and still innocent. My home was about an hour-and-a-half drive from the hospital where I was studying, and sometimes I went there for the weekend. While there, I would talk to my parents about my experiences caring for patients at the hospital. I was in my first year of nursing, eager to learn, and doing a practicum on a medical/surgical unit. This included interacting with patients, assisting with personal care, checking vital signs, and doing post-operative care.

I remember one patient assignment, a middle-aged man who was short and bald, with a heavy-set frame. The report I got was that he was quite independent, able to get out of bed on his own, and do his own personal care. After I checked his vital signs, he told me he was going to get up to go to the bathroom. I could see by the look on his face that he was in quite a bit of pain.

With one sweep of his arm, he pulled the sheets off his body in order to set his legs free to emerge and set his feet to the floor. Standing at the foot of the bed, I couldn't believe my eyes. He was wearing only a johnny shirt [hospital gown] his privates were completely exposed. His legs looked very far apart. There, in full view, was a gigantic scrotum. It was at least the size of his head. It was extremely large, pale, and shiny. I didn't think this was normal, but at that time I had only seen the private parts of babies and children when I changed their diapers or helped with toileting and dressing when I was baby-sitting. I felt sad for this patient as he was extremely uncomfortable. It turned out that he had "hydrocele testes," which is a pathological accumulation of serous fluid in his scrotum. It can occur for many different reasons, such as cancer, infection, and trauma. I was shocked.

When I told this story to my parents, they were speechless. I don't think they really knew what to say to relax me. No doubt they were quite aware that this new and unsettling experience was only the first of many that I would encounter during my career. Of course, they were right.

MARIAN FACCIOLO

Can I Check Your Dressing?
Kelly M.'s Story

I had been working as registered nurse for only a couple of years and will always remember this one incident.

I was working on a surgical unit. It was early on in my shift. I reviewed the cardex for information on all my patients in order to plan and organize my workload for the shift. After doing this, I went in to see a couple of my male patients who occupied a semi-private room. Both were post-operative. One of them had a hernia repair and the other had a circumcision.

I went to the bedside of one of the men and asked if I could check his penis. He seemed surprised and uncomfortable as he looked up at me standing beside him. It was obvious he wasn't accustomed to having to show this part of his anatomy to strangers, and certainly not to a young shameless nurse. He did comply and showed me his penis. There was nothing post-operative about it.

I felt very embarrassed and speechless as I retreated from his room. As it turned out, it was his roommate who had the circumcision, and he was the one with the hernia repair. Both needed to have their post-op areas checked. I just had the patients mixed up.

The lesson I learned that day was to always say "Can I check your dressing?" This would be vague enough for further investigation and save me from any more of these embarrassing situations. I guess I could also check their name bands, too.

FRONT LINE NURSING STORIES

I Took a Refresher Course
Rosa's Story

I had just returned to work after a four-month refresher course because I had left nursing for a few years.

I was working on availability at a large hospital, and back in those days they sent you to work on any unit that was short of nurses. So, one Saturday, I was sent to a urology floor. I had never worked on a surgical urology unit. Being the eager nurse that I was, with my recent refresher courses and emergency training, I went to the unit with confidence that I would be able to handle any situation on this floor.

It was seven-thirty in the morning, and the nurse in charge gave me the list of patients I would be taking care of that shift. I was sitting at the desk, reviewing the charts, when another nurse pointed out one of my patients. Mr. X. was walking down the hall. I turned around and looked at him. I quickly assessed that he was an elderly, frail man walking in a slow, shuffling manner while holding on to his Foley catheter. I continued to look at him until I saw his backside. His johnny shirt was open at the back, exposing his derriere, and I could see he had a very large bandage between his legs. I deduced that he'd had surgery along his perineum. The charge nurse confirmed that "Yes, he had a scrotum lift"!

I was thinking, "Oh! What is that?" as I continued looking at his back. Then I noted, with my eagle eyes, a trace of blood going down his left leg. Being the vigilant nurse that I thought I was, I asked myself, "What is the first thing you do when there is bleeding?"

I immediately put my hand behind him, applying pressure while lifting his testicles as he walked down the hall. I noted that he suddenly started walking quite fast, though it still seemed like an eternity until we got to his room. I helped him sit on the edge of his bed.

He looked at me with an annoyed manner and said, "What is going on here?"

I said, "Sir, you are bleeding where you were operated on, and I must evaluate the problem."

He turned around on the bed. I removed the bandage and realized that it was just some old blood from before, nothing to worry about. I was content that I had done a very good job... until I shared this adventure with my husband!

What a day it was! Now I know how to motivate elderly men to walk.

Sex and Back Pain
Valerie's Story

Like most of my class, I had my bags all packed and ready to go to Texas, as jobs in Ontario were scarce in 1977. A week before my flight to Houston, I received a job offer from a hospital in Toronto, which I accepted, because I had a boyfriend here.

The floor I was working on had forty medical beds with nine psych beds. Interestingly, about eighty percent of our patients spoke Portuguese, and I spoke only English. You can imagine that the therapeutic nursing interventions were less than ideal.

Two of the patients, Paula and Jake, had struck up a friendship and spent all their time together. She was nineteen and married, and Jake was forty-five and married, but not to Paula. I don't remember her issue. He was in hospital with intractable back pain. The doctors could not find a physical reason for it. He had a claim in for Workman's Compensation with regards to his back.

At the time of the incident, I was on midnights and making my rounds. I went into Paula's room, but she wasn't there. I continued my rounds and found her in Jake's room. They were having sex. He was on top and moving very well for someone who could barely move because of his pain.

I have since learned that just because you have back pain, it doesn't necessarily mean that sex is not an option. But I was young and judgmental, probably more because of the age difference than anything, and even though she was married... she was only nineteen!

I continued my rounds. I did not say anything to them. I stewed about it during the night. What is my responsibility? Was it any of my business?

On my final rounds I went into his room, not sure what I was going to say. (Why did I think I had to say anything?) What came out of my mouth was, "I saw you last night with Paula, and you certainly didn't look like your back was bothering you!" Then I stalked out of the room. I reported the incident to the supervisor before going home in the morning.

I got a call around suppertime as I was getting ready for work. It was the supervisor, telling me that it was best for me to work on a different floor for a couple of days as the male patient was threatening to "kill that nurse who had ratted on him." I guess the psychiatrist came in and read him the riot act, and his claim for Workman's Compensation was being re-examined. I worked the next night on a different floor, and Jake was discharged the next day. I think Paula was also discharged home. Hence, I could go back to my regular floor.

Things that I have learned since then:
- Sex is sometimes good for back pain.
- It is not okay to threaten your nurse's life, no matter what.
- What I feel about something doesn't always have to be shared with the world.
- Make more noise when entering a patient's room.

Val is quite clear about what she has learned. She recognizes that she was upset about the age difference and how her own judgment about certain things played into her response. I believe her upset led her to report the incident.

MARIAN FACCIOLO

Lessons Learned as a Student
Karen's Story

As a nursing student, I worked summers in a chronic care facility. I was young, naïve, and idealistic, and these summers gave me a dose of reality. One of the units where I was frequently assigned had many young males who were paraplegic or quadriplegic. Many of their injuries were the result of high-risk behaviours involving drugs or alcohol or both. I found that for many of these young men, their accidents didn't change their lifestyles. Rather, they became less concerned with the consequences. They had already experienced the worst-case scenario, so being cautious and conservative didn't mean much at that point.

As a young nursing student who also happened to blush very easily, I was an easy target for their jokes and pranks. I was asked to "adjust" more than a few genitals, some of them clearly in working order. We had the occasional drug raid by police with their dogs, and Saturday night sometimes meant helping an intoxicated, stoned resident into bed. As a unit, we had many discussions about respecting residents' lifestyle choices non-judgmentally, which was sometimes hard to do. As unpredictable as that unit was, I really enjoyed working there, and not much shocked me after that!

FRONT LINE NURSING STORIES

From the Community to the Emergency Department
Debbie's Story

Debbie, an ER nurse, told me that she was surprised at the many issues nurses in the community must deal with.

I was a staff nurse in the hospital trauma bay emergency department. An elderly lady was brought into the unit. After she came in, the whole ER department smelled like rotting carcass. Two generators were required to deal with the odour.

The scenario was pieced together later.

This elderly lady had been living with her elderly husband. He had mild to moderate dementia. The lady had diabetes. Her husband had called the local community agency, where all the new community referrals are directed. He told them he needed help because he could not get his wife out of the chair any longer. Usually they arrange to have a case manager do an initial home visit to do a complete and thorough assessment. In this case, they decided to send in a visiting nurse prior to this. The husband sounded quite distressed, and it was thought that they needed a nurse to visit in the home as soon as possible. By talking with the husband, who was the referral source, it was evident that something was wrong, but he was not able to provide some important information. The husband was compromised cognitively, but he was doing what he could to help his wife. There were no family or close friends available for support.

The nurse went into the home. As the husband opened the door, she could smell a very putrid odour of decay. She thought the person was dead, as the odour was so overpoweringly bad.

The nurse who made the visit discovered that the lady had been sitting in a wicker chair. She could not ambulate to the toilet or anywhere else. In order to try to relieve her discomfort, her spouse had cut a hole in the chair for her to void and have a bowel movement. The lady was found to have become necrotic from the waist down. The nurse was shocked that she was still alive. When taken off the chair, her skin remained on the seat. She lasted maybe a day after being admitted to hospital.

It drove home to me that these patients can be in the community and can be totally isolated and missed. The neighbours and family did not know the situation that the couple were living in. They had no formal help in the home, and no one other than the husband was there regularly. His health was compromised. As far as he knew, he was doing what he could to help her situation.

One of My First Night Shifts
Marina's Story

When I started nursing, I thought it would be interesting. As my career progressed, nursing developed into something more than I ever could have imagined. At the end of the day, I feel positive. I believe that what you get out of nursing depends on your perspective, your experiences, and the type of person you are.

I was working on a medical/surgical unit. I remember a young woman who was admitted from eastern Canada somewhere. When I say young, she was in her mid-fifties. I say she was young as she was too young to be dying. I met her on the night shift. Her room was dimly lit. I tiptoed around her bed. I didn't want to wake her with a bright light, so I was careful not to shine the flashlight in her face. The nurse from the previous shift reported that this lady had been in severe pain from the time of admission the day before.

As I approached her, I felt a cool calmness in her presence. Her husband entered the room. What does a person say in this type of situation? I didn't say anything. He told me that their children had just left before I came in.

He was struggling. She was struggling. Here I was at work, standing at her bedside, and I felt like we were the only three people on earth.

I lifted her arm to wrap the blood pressure cuff around it. The material of the cuff brushed over the large cauliflower-like chest tumour that protruded from her body. As I did this, I felt a bit queasy as I thought of the growth that was proliferating beneath, that was ravaging her body at places within, draining the life from her without regard for anything or anyone. She was literally decaying before our eyes. I stepped in front of her husband to shield his view, completed my assessment, and left the room.

A few days later, the woman passed away. There was talk about how she did not want chemotherapy. She had travelled out east to be treated naturally with some alternative medicine. Health care professionals spoke of her options and her treatment decisions. I watched her young adult children and husband leave their mother and wife behind. At this time I was a very new and "green" nurse. As time passes and these types of experiences accumulate, you change. I don't think I have ever hugged my mom as hard as I did the next time I saw her after that experience.

This novice nurse is trying to work through her own feelings about dealing with death and dying. The wound area itself is foreign and disturbing to her. She becomes acutely aware of her own vulnerability and has a glimpse of just how fragile and mortal we all are. Marina is a nurse, but she is also a woman who has a mother of her own whom she loves.

MARIAN FACCIOLO

Nobody Should Be in this Type of Pain When Dying
Marian's Story

The year was 1974. I was the nurse in charge on a private medical/surgical floor at a general hospital in the city of Montreal. Because it was a private floor, we had both medical and surgical patients and covered a wide variety of conditions. We served people of all ages on that ward. The key word was "private," so the patients on this floor either had money or private insurance or both.

I recall one of these patients very well. Edith was a single lady in her sixties. She had cancer of the breast with metastasis. I remember her because there were two things that stood out during the time she was a patient on our floor. The first thing was that she had very few friends or family. As a matter of fact, during my shifts working with her, she had no visitors except one. Her friend was also single and about the same age. The friend was a nurse who worked in our hospital in an administration role. This meant that Edith spent many hours alone.

I recall an evening when I was working. Edith was in tremendous pain. Generally, she presented as very stoic. That evening, I was acutely aware of her agony. She would let out these blood-curdling cries, almost as if she was being tortured. They came in waves. She had received her prescribed pain medication, but this time it wasn't working. Enough time had passed, and the medication should have taken effect.

The doctor in charge of her care was summoned to the ward. He was a well-respected physician at our hospital. I was at the desk and saw him wandering down the hall to see Edith. On his return he called me into the treatment room. It was as if he had a big secret to share. He told me that he needed to help Edith and wanted me to go down to the labour and delivery room and sign out one heroin tablet. It was not a drug used often but was one of the medications kept in the labour and delivery room and counted there. He called the unit ahead, and they were expecting me when I arrived.

Although quite surprised, I followed the staff doctor's direction and returned promptly to the ward, where he anxiously waited for me. He guided me back to the treatment room, where he pulled out a Bunsen burner and a spoon. He lit the burner with a match and dissolved the heroin in normal saline on the spoon. He asked me to hold the spoon while he drew up the medication with a needle and syringe. He looked at me as if this was something secretive that he wanted kept quiet. I don't remember him saying anything, but just the way he looked at me—it was as if this would be our little pact. I felt there was a non-verbal agreement on my part, and I was now a partner in crime.

Once the syringe was loaded, he turned and walked down the corridor to administer some much-needed relief to Edith. It wasn't long before she gained relief from her misery. There were no more cries. The doctor broke protocol and she finally slept.

I can never forget how the mercy of one physician played a significant role in providing her some comfort during her darkest hours. Don't forget, this was a long time ago, and pain management has improved drastically since then. Pain management is key for palliative patients, and Edith was deemed palliative.

This doctor and I never spoke of this event. No one ever questioned me about it. I felt relief for Edith. She was not long for this world after that, and I don't recall a time when she was again in such pain.

I know this physician was well ahead of his time. Palliative care now is not what it was forty-five years ago. If a physician does not know how to adequately assist with pain control, then it is in the patient's best interest to make a referral to one who does. There are also pain specialists and palliative care physicians who can be consulted. Palliative care has become a specialty. Nurses who work in this area usually have added knowledge, skills, and experience to facilitate pain and symptom management, planning, and better outcomes when possible.

MARIAN FACCIOLO

Labour and Delivery Twins Discovered
Marian's Story

I was working the day shift in obstetrics, which at the time was referred to as the "case room." It was in a city hospital that did a significant number of deliveries each year.

I had only been working in labour and delivery for about a year and a half, so I still considered myself to be a novice nurse. This was a specialty area and there was a lot to learn before I could consider myself an expert.

I was assigned to admit and care for a lady who had just walked into the unit at the change of shift. I did the usual assessment and gathered the pertinent data. Part of my routine was to do the Leopold manoeuvre. I had learned this as part of my obstetrics course. It wasn't a mandatory procedure. The lady I had just admitted had a very large abdomen, but so do many others. I listened to the fetal heart. I then did the manoeuvre, which consists of a process of laying one's hands on the woman's abdomen to gently palpate the position of the baby. There is a series of four specific steps in palpating the uterus through the abdomen in order to determine the lie and presentation of the fetus.

Once I finished doing the procedure, I was quite sure I could feel two babies. I then listened to the fetal heart again and checked for a fetal heart where I thought the other baby was lying. Sure enough, I could hear another fetal heart. Sometimes this can be tricky, as the sound of one heart can be heard in different areas of the abdomen. In any case, the second heart rate was a different rate from the other.

I went out of the patient's room to the nurse's station, where the head nurse was standing talking with my patient's obstetrician. He had just arrived on the unit. I told them what I had found. An ultrasound confirmed that there were twins. At the time, ultrasounds were not done on a routine basis.

I was happy to have been able to make this kind of contribution. I think everyone was better able to deal with the trajectory of this lady's labour and delivery with this extremely valuable information.

It was a confidence booster for me. As long as I worked in the case room, I always did the Leopold manoeuvre. It helped me diagnose a longitudinal lie and breech presentations. It is so non-invasive and provides a wealth of information.

Meditation, Labour, and Birth
Marian's Story

Near the end of my day shift, an Indian lady came into the labour and delivery room. Montreal is a multicultural community, and this was a busy obstetrical centre. The patient was dressed in a traditional sari, had a bindi on her forehead, and spoke English. She was alone and in early labour. I did the admission and settled her into the room.

After checking on my other patients, I returned to see how she was progressing. When I opened the door, I was taken aback! The patient was sitting upright, cross-legged, on the bed with the white top sheet covering her entire body. This unfamiliar sight caught me off guard. I didn't know what to think. What was this all about?

She informed me that she was meditating. This was how she was going to work through her labour. It served her well, because she was completely under control with each contraction. I had never seen this before and must admit that it felt strange to be in this unfamiliar territory.

Soon, my shift ended. I gave a report to the two nurses coming on the evening shift and went home.

The next day, I got a report on the Indian lady whom I had met the previous day. Apparently she managed extremely well up to and including the delivery of the baby. She meditated during her labour and delivered a healthy, good-sized baby. Everything had gone as expected.

The nurse giving the report then became emotional and sounded distraught! As she told it, everything went well until the fourth stage of labour. This last stage includes the first four hours after the baby is delivered. In this stage, the mom is monitored closely to be sure that she voids, that there is no excess bleeding, and that vital signs are normal.

The lady was fine initially, but when the nurse returned to check ten to fifteen minutes later, she was unable to get a blood pressure reading. There was a faint sound. The pulse was rapid and "thread-like." There was no response from the patient. The nurse prodded her and called her name. Her colour was very pale. Her uterus wasn't palpable. She was hemorrhaging vaginally.

The nurse sounded an alarm, and the nurse's co-worker and the resident who delivered the baby rushed to her side. Everyone was upset and beside themselves. There was already an intravenous set up, because at that time it was standard procedure to have one in place at the time of delivery. The IV flow was increased, and the uterus was massaged. Medication was added to the IV. Still, she did not respond.

With continued intervention by the doctor and nurse, the patient finally responded. They were able to communicate with her. Finally, the situation was under control. They saved her life.

Later, when she was stable and before she was transferred to her room on the floor, the woman told them about her own experience during this ordeal. She told them that she had continued to meditate during the fourth stage. She told them that while the emergency was happening, she felt her spirit hovering over her body. She watched them in their panic-stricken state. She watched as they repeatedly took her blood pressure and pulse, called her name, massaged her uterus, added medication to the IV, and increased the intravenous fluids. She watched while the staff shook with fear. She watched as their anxiety skyrocketed and they rushed to do all they could to save her life. Her spirit hovered over their care and concern while her body lay there, almost lifeless. She told them that she felt sorry for all of them. She felt especially sorry for the resident, who thought he was going to lose her. She told them that she felt their pain and their concern and so decided to come back. She vividly expressed what she had observed and felt while they rescued her from near death.

As nurses, we are continually learning. Working with this lady, it became clear to me that I did not know much about Indian culture. I did not know much about meditation and alternative ways of dealing with pain. I had done yoga, but this was at a different level. My experience, and that of my colleagues, gave me a wake-up call. For me, it solidified the need to keep my eyes and ears open, ask questions, share valuable information, and continue to learn about people and culture.

Prolapsed Cord
Marian's Story

I was a labour and delivery room nurse. It was the change of shift from evenings to nights. At the time, we had a buddy system and usually worked with the same co-workers for night shifts. For the evenings, there were two nurses who usually worked together on the same rotation. We referred to them as "the two Judys."

My buddy and I arrived at the front desk, ready to get the evening report. This time, things were different. Sometimes it can get hectic, but tonight it was chaos. The two Judys were rushing and scurrying. It was obviously a crisis. They had already placed an emergency call to the resident physician, the obstetrician, and the anesthesiologist.

The pregnant lady who was under their charge was lying in the hospital bed with the foot of the bed elevated. They had already moved the patient to the front desk, where report is given. Nurse Judy was kneeling on the bottom part of the bed. She had her hand, or at least several of her fingers, in the patient's vagina while she shouted orders. Her voice was shaky. She told me to run and get a sterile cloth soaked in saline to wrap around the baby's umbilical cord. I ran for the towel, put on sterile gloves, wet the towel, and brought it, along with the rest of the saline, to the patient's bed. I wrapped the wet towel around the umbilical cord, which I could now see was hanging out between the patient's legs. Judy continued to hold her fingers in place to keep the baby's presenting part from pressing too hard against the cord and cutting off the blood flow and oxygenation to the baby's vital organs.

The patient in the bed was quiet. I could never recall her face or anything she said during this emergency. I do remember the second Judy at the head of the bed and me at the foot of the bed. We were moving the bed down the hall to get to the operating room. These beds can be heavy to push. It must have been the adrenaline because I don't remember the "heavy" part. We were pushing not only the patient in the bed but also the other Judy, who managed to keep this baby getting vital oxygen until the Caesarian section was done.

Not every day in labour and delivery is this dramatic, but I do believe we worked as a team to save this baby's life. Judy said that when the lady's water broke, she did an internal examination and found the cord coming out. She knew it was a medical emergency, and everyone knew to do their part. We were all aware of the potential for tragic results.

In this emergency, I learned how vital it is to understand the normal birthing process in order to recognize and successfully intervene in critical situations. It is also important to understand potential adverse conditions. The two nurses who were initially involved recognized the acuity and severity of the event. They provided lifesaving emergency measures to save this baby and prevent a catastrophe. During this delivery, the entire team brought their skills to bear to prevent a tragedy.

FRONT LINE NURSING STORIES

Patients Know a Lot About Themselves
Deirdre's Story

Beth has lived most of her life in an institution for people with developmental disabilities. She is in a wheelchair and cannot talk. I first met her when she was fifty-five, after she had been diagnosed with Type I diabetes. She received insulin daily. Her caregivers had been taught that she must follow a strict diet in order to keep her glucose levels in range.

Over time, Beth began to refuse to eat any food. She would turn her head and strike out at anyone who tried to feed her. The staff became very distressed. They knew the importance of ensuring that Beth ate regularly. They expressed fear that Beth would go into a diabetic coma and die if she did not eat. They thought that Beth was refusing to eat because she was becoming senile. They did not believe that Beth understood the connection between taking insulin injections and eating.

We held a series of case conferences to find ways to support Beth. The physician, psychologist, dietitian, and I developed strategies that would help the staff manage her food intake.

The staff tried everything. One day, Beth's blood sugar dropped dangerously low and she was sent to the hospital by ambulance. While in hospital, the physicians discovered that Beth's esophagus was almost completely closed over. It seems that Beth also had GERD (gastric esophageal reflux disease). GERD is a condition where hydrochloric acid from the stomach splashes up into the esophagus. This splashing causes heartburn. As Beth was unable to speak, she was not able to tell anyone about the discomfort caused by the heartburn.

To make matters worse, the chronic splashing of hydrochloric acid had scarred the esophagus to a point that food could not pass from the esophagus into the stomach. While we were worried that Beth would have a diabetic reaction because she wasn't eating, Beth was trying to tell us that food was piling up in her esophagus and she was choking. Beth's ordeal ended when she received a gastrostomy tube that allowed food to pass directly into the stomach.

We, her care team, felt terrible. We were so focused on the fact that she needed nutrition after receiving insulin that we stopped listening to her when she tried to tell us that eating was dangerous for her. We assumed that she was incapable of understanding the consequences of not eating. We never once thought that perhaps she knew what was best for her. We only had to listen.

One of the things nurses come to understand is that patients often know much more about themselves, their bodies, and their situations than we sometimes give them credit for. Deirdre speaks about this aspect when she tells us of Beth's health and healing process.

In the Community

Over the years, the settings and roles for nurses have expanded. They have gone from the hospital to home care and to various community environments that exist to support health care: schools, family health teams, health clinics (diabetic and chronic illness), shelters and drop-in centres, and more. In the next story, I describe some of what's involved in community nursing.

Community Nursing
Marian's Story

For the most part, I had worked in the acute care setting of a Montreal hospital. I had enjoyed my time there and learned a lot. First, I worked on a medical/surgical private floor. This was great, as I got a lot of broad experience. Then I moved to labour and delivery and then to hemodialysis. The last two specialty areas were great, and once again, I learned a lot.

FRONT LINE NURSING STORIES

At some point in the mid-1980s, my husband's job took us to Ontario. I worked as a casual in the local hospital while taking a neonatal intensive care course in Toronto at the Hospital for Sick Children. While doing this, I applied for and obtained a job working as a visiting nurse in the community. I filled in for district nurses when they were off and then had a district of my own. I thoroughly enjoyed the work. I remember being quite surprised at the difference between hospital and community work.

In the community, it felt like I was so much more on my own. There were policies and procedures, as in the hospital, but there was much more independence. I had peers, but everyone was as busy as I was, and there was not a lot of chance to commiserate over problems or issues. There were no physicians physically in the area who I could discuss medical issues with. The nurses in community could call the patient's doctor and leave messages or request a call back to discuss things. The doctors were busy in their offices, seeing patients themselves.

Another significant thing about working in the community is that I was providing medical support in the patients' domain. Although in the hospital the patient was the centre of care, moving to the community gave a whole new meaning to this. I was now on their turf, and patients were the captain of their own ship. It was very positive for patients. In the hospital, it was usually the patient with whom I communicated. Of course, I spoke with the family too when they were visiting. But I got to see much more of the family when doing home visiting. I worked more intensely with both the patient and the family. I continued to teach, do the procedures, and do relationship building, but now there were more people to work with.

It was a whole new learning experience to get to know people in their own environment. People's environments were as different as the people themselves. I liked it. At times, though, it could be really challenging. As a nurse, there was so much more information available to better understand the person in their everyday environment.

As a district nurse, I planned my own day and the day of whoever was working with me in my area. The agency I worked with in the community had what is called "time per visit." They kept track of how many visits a nurse did in a day. I learned that there were some visits that were quick and easy, and others that would be much more time-consuming. Did it make one nurse better than another because one could see seven people a day and another could see ten or more? Palliative care patients usually required more time. More complex patients required more time. The geography that needed to be covered and the time for travel needed to be taken into consideration. Doing a dressing can be a short and quick visit compared to providing palliation at home with a patient who needs pain control and a family that needs teaching. Patient acuity and complexity make a difference in time and effort required to provide nursing care. I don't believe this aspect was given enough consideration. I saw excellent nurses being called into the office to have their time per visit discussed. I believed that there needed to be a way to ensure the job got done well without demoralizing some of the people doing the job. Productivity and patient outcomes should be evaluated using a multipronged approach.

One of the things I learned was how to communicate with the case manager who I worked and conferenced with regularly. I learned to work more independently and know who I could rely on as my buddy in the community. I learned when the physician really needed to be called. I learned that patients and their families are all so different. I got a whole lot more information when I could see and appreciate patients in their own environment. I got a better appreciation of what district or community nurses do and the challenges they are up against, trying their best to get the job done. Over the years, as I changed jobs and became a case manager, I saw the expansion of the visiting nurses' scope of practice and an increase in the acuity and complexity of patients. More and more knowledge and skills were required, and more demands were placed on the visiting nurses.

Preparedness
Mary's Story

I was the night shift nurse working in the home of a thirty-year-old man with cancer of the heart muscle. He had been diagnosed only three months earlier.

The patient was married with three children. He had two daughters, eight and ten years of age, and a six-year-old son. Working the night shift, I never got to meet his children until the last night.

Every night, I would care for him while his wife slept next to him. She would either share his bed or sleep on a small cot set up beside him. He had a hospital bed. It was very crowded, with three large, soft Gund animals. He always wanted them close to him.

I could see and feel the love the couple shared. On the last night, the wife informed me that they had decided she should try to get a good night's sleep in another room. I was to wake her if he wanted or needed her. They kissed good night and said they loved each other.

It was a little after four a.m. when he sat up and had a grape popsicle. I administered his pain medication, rubbed his back and pressure points, made him comfortable. He took my hand in his and thanked me. He closed his eyes and slept. Within the hour, he had slipped away.

I called the family physician and woke his wife up. She quickly came to his room and stayed with him for about ten minutes. Then she went upstairs to wake the children.

The doctor arrived. I soon realized she had developed a great relationship with this family. She hugged each of them. She had fully prepared the family for this night. Each of the children went up to their dad. One by one they kissed him and told him they loved him. One by one they each took one of the stuffed animals away with them.

The doctor explained that earlier in the disease process, the children had gone to the store. With their mother's help, each of them chose a special stuffed animal to give to their dad. The plan was that he would give the stuffed animals back to them after he passed away. The stuffed animals now had their dad's "smell" on them. They each retrieved their gift and hugged and held the animal close. There were no tears except for my own. I quickly wiped them away.

The kids went downstairs to sit at the dining room table. They each wrote a special letter for their dad to take with him. They took their time. They wrote their letters and drew special pictures to give as gifts for their dad. Mom gave them letters that dad had written for each of them.

The funeral home arrived to take his body to the morgue. The children were prepared for each step of what was happening. The patient's wife told me that the physician had sat all of them down and explained everything that was going to happen. The patient was there as well. There were no surprises, no whispering behind their backs. The whole family had been involved with everything along the way.

I finished my nursing documentation and said my goodbyes. I left the home, knowing that even though the family had suffered a tragedy and would continue to grieve for their husband and father, the situation was made easier because of a kind, caring doctor who had taken the time to prepare this family.

I know transitions can be difficult. I have worked hard in my career to help patients through them. On this day, I was reminded that as health care professionals we can and do make a difference in both the process and the outcome. In this case, with this patient and family, I believe that the physician was able to facilitate movement through the dying process. I learned from her. I was able to transfer some of these attitudes and beliefs to other care situations. Each patient and family is different. Each scenario is different and very much affected by the values, belief systems, readiness and culture of the people involved. On this day, I understood the value of preparing people as best you can and as much as they will allow.

FRONT LINE NURSING STORIES

A Hoarder
Lois's Story

One day I got a telephone call from Lily, who was Mary's friend. She called to say Mary couldn't get up off the couch anymore and that she wanted to go to the hospital. Mary never returned home again, as a nursing home bed was found for her.

I first met Mary when I did the initial assessment visit at her home. She was a ninety-year-old retired nurse who had trouble with her heart. She had fluid on her lungs from congestive heart failure. A visiting nurse was needed to teach her how to manage her heart failure, ensure she took her medication, and limit her salt and water intake. When meeting her, I realized she had been lying on her couch all day and all night. Her legs were very swollen and heavy. Working as a case manager in the community, one of my roles was to negotiate with my patients and try to improve safety and chronic disease management while the person stayed at home. At my first visit, Mary told me that she didn't ever want to leave her home.

It was obvious that Mary had a problem with hoarding. When I entered her home, there was a pathway through the paper, boxes, and clothes piled two feet high on either side. I tried to interest Mary in allowing the papers and boxes to be removed, little by little, to allow more room for her walker. That was not something Mary wanted to do. She made it very clear to me that the papers and newspapers were there waiting for her to feel better. She told me that when she felt better, she would organize them into a collection and decide what she should keep and what she could dispose of. She didn't want to leave her home, but didn't know what the future might hold. She had lived there forever, many years alone, and previously with her mother before she died.

She told me she couldn't afford to pay a cleaning woman to help her with the housework because she had "no money for that anymore." She said she had hired a contractor who had ripped her off. He had been paid in full, but had not finished the job. She focused on the dishonesty of this man, who talked her into a repair of her roof and siding but left the work unfinished. It was as if this had happened a few days ago, but I soon realized it had occurred several years earlier—and she had never gotten over it.

She loved cats and bought big bags of cat food to feed all the strays in the neighbourhood. She had about eight to ten cats visiting every morning. She had an old tabby cat indoors, too. That tabby was thin and old, and Mary allowed her to stay in the house. When I visited, she insisted I put down a towel to sit on, so I didn't get cat hair on my clothes.

My attempt to interest Mary in clearing out her home so she could be safer was futile. I did talk her into allowing a social worker to help her make some plans for a power of attorney (POA) and get her finances in order. She confided that she hadn't filed income taxes for several years.

It was out of the question to ask a personal support worker (PSW) to try to work on the papers. Mary said she would only allow a PSW to feed her cats and heat up some TV dinners. She made her trip to the bathroom several times a day and told me she could wash herself at the sink if needed. There was no way she could bathe in the tub, because it was full of clothes and cardboard.

A few weeks after the nursing visits started, I was told there was a flea infestation in the house, and the nurses couldn't visit unless the house was fumigated. I told Mary this, but she would only agree to ask Lily to buy some spray to use on the furniture. The floors were covered with paper and couldn't be sprayed.

The social worker had started to visit and thought she was making headway by helping to get Mary's income taxes done. There were discussions about which relative she would ask to take her POA. She had alienated all but three of them, her sister's children. She had decided to ask them to help. Given Mary's age, medical status, home situation, and risks, it was important for the POA to be in place.

Between us, the social worker and I reasoned with Mary and convinced her to apply to a nursing home. We said this was just in case she needed it one day. She reluctantly agreed that she was getting too frail to stay alone in her home. She realized that only Lily, her cousin's widow, was interested in helping her, and Lily had limited time to spend with her. She told us she had no one else who would venture into her house, because it was so cluttered.

The last time I visited her, I met her friend Lily in the doorway. Mary was lying on the couch, and things looked pretty much the same as the previous time I had visited. Mary had signed her nursing home choice list, and we chatted briefly about what she should do with all the stuff she hadn't yet looked at. She said her old tabby cat had died, and she could only get her cat fix when she opened the door to feed the strays. The local paper came daily. She had a magnifying glass that she used to read it. She had cut out some articles of interest and said she thought she would read them later when she felt up to it. She asked me to come in for a visit and a cup of tea. I said I couldn't that day, but maybe some other time. The truth was that I really didn't want to sit down in that flea-infested room, but I felt so guilty about this fact that I just said, "Another time." My response was met with a smile and, "I'll look forward to that."

As I walked to the car, I thought about why she kept all that stuff around her. I realized that the hoarding of all those articles and old clothes was a long-time habit of putting things off until later, when she felt more energetic. I hope I won't be like her in my old age, sitting on my couch, watching for stray cats, reading the daily paper with a magnifying glass, and talking on the phone to whoever calls. I hope I have more in my life when I am weak and frail. I hope I have friends and family who will still come by for a visit. I hope I won't be all alone with my things piled all around me.

I guess what Mary taught me is that one's home is precious. No one else can understand what happy and sad events took place within those walls: memories of a much happier time, of family meals, happy laughter, and lots of conversations with loved ones. The thought occurred to me that health care professionals come into people's homes and sometimes try to make them what they should be, safer and more convenient.

Home sweet home is what Mary had until she had to leave it. I will never forget Mary. She taught me a lot. Keep what you want to keep as long as it can be used and you can still walk around safely. Don't give up your independence. And above all, read whatever you can read for as long as you can, even if it means using a magnifying glass.

MARIAN FACCIOLO

I Do and I Will
Nichole's Story

I was working as a case manager in 2001, my first year working with a particular community agency. I worked on the Adult Program. At that time, our model was such that we did both a placement component and an in-home service component. Our assessments were still done on paper, not computers. It was a general model, and I had adults of all ages and stages of life, including palliative care.

The couple I visited that day were probably among the first seniors I visited in my new role. It was one of my first times doing placement. This was a reassessment visit.

The wife had personal support in place a couple of times a week for bathing. She was diagnosed with Alzheimer's disease. They lived in a small bungalow on a beautiful piece of property, in a rural area of the county. It was springtime. There were beautiful lilacs and other flowers in the yard. The property was so lush. As I drove up to the house, I felt a quiet sense of peace and tranquility.

An elderly gentleman, the spouse, dressed in an Easter egg–blue suit, greeted me at the door. You could tell that he'd probably had that suit for most of his life and wore it on special occasions such as this. You could tell that the couple probably didn't get much company. He brought me into the living room and introduced me to his wife. She too was in her late eighties, a couple of years older than him. She was the patient, and she was cognitively impaired. She sat in a wheelchair, dressed in a lovely dress and pantyhose, and was impeccably groomed. I spent time talking with her, and it was evident that her dementia was advanced. She didn't make much sense. She pointed to the birds outside. However, she seemed to enjoy our interaction.

I was surprised that they were managing so well under the circumstances. The house was clean, and nothing seemed out of place. There were no reports from caregivers indicating that the couple were not coping, even though she required a high level of personal care and supervision in order to be effectively supported at home. I spent time talking with them and getting to know both. She wasn't mobilizing well, and he was her caregiver.

I completed the assessment. I wanted to get an idea of how they were managing, and I mentioned that if there was a day he couldn't manage and needed more help, then he could call me. After all, he was the main caregiver, and they did not have any family support. I was concerned that he would eventually break down and might need to have her placed in a nursing home.

I brought up the notion of placement. Thinking about the interaction still brings tears to my eyes. He said to me, "Sixty-five years ago I said I do, and I will."

He thanked me for my time. I was struck by his feelings, his commitment to his wife. She was so happy in her environment. It was obvious to me that she had her needs met. He was committed to this. He was devoted to her and committed to their life together. It spoke to his values and relationships. She was very content and was thriving in her own environment and in the relationship. It changed, or at least strengthened, the way I looked at relationships, commitments, and marriage. At the time, I remember being in a relationship and engaged to the man I later married. I will never forget this couple. I was inspired by them and their relationship and their commitment to each other. They were happy together.

In nursing, we have many opportunities to learn about relationships, both good and bad, as many of these stories indicate. In situations where the patient has strong support, whether from a spouse, a family member or friends, the healing process is made easier. There is no substitute for strong informal support that stems from love.

MARIAN FACCIOLO

God and Hope
Marian's Story

I was working as a community case manager. I received a new referral for a patient named Carol who lived with her daughter. Carol had several adult children and a few grandchildren. Whenever she spoke of the grandkids, she beamed.

Carol had been diagnosed with metastatic ovarian cancer several years prior to this. The trajectory of her disease had been a long road of illness and many treatments. This time, we were involved because she had been in a Toronto hospital for brain surgery and radiation. On admission to our program, she required nursing care and personal support.

When I made the first home visit, I found Carol to be lethargic. She was in a hospital bed and was quite limited in her mobility and ambulation. There was a walker in place, and bath aids. She required assistance for transfers, personal care, and toileting. Personal support workers provided help with these activities of daily living. Nursing was involved for monitoring, care for her wound, and pain and symptom management. Carol's daughter needed some respite care.

On the day of my visit, her daughter provided most of the information, as Carol was too tired and drowsy. I understood that this was related to the brain traumas she had recently undergone. Although she was palliative, I was not sure what to expect as to her prognosis. I completed the assessment. Her function was poor. She had just returned home after completing radiation treatment at the hospital and radiation took its toll.

About three weeks later, reports from the nurses in the home indicated that Carol was improving significantly. Both her mobility and cognition were better. I decided to make another home visit. This time, Carol was much more alert. We were able to converse, and subsequently, I got to know her better. I discovered that she was full of life. She was able to discuss her disease and family situation openly and honestly. She wanted me to get to know her, and I enjoyed this opportunity. Although she had been sick for several years, Carol continued to be optimistic and at the same time realistic about her prognosis.

The reason I remember her so well is that she was different from many other palliative patients I had met. Two things struck me about Carol. One was the way she spoke with me about her deep faith in God. Her faith was her anchor. She was also religious and attended church regularly. The other was that she was very positive about her situation. Her family physician and specialists had informed her of the disease and what she could expect all the way along. She had her own expectation of her situation, and she was extremely hopeful. It was as if she took in what she was told, valued that input, but also took charge of what she could do herself. Carol told me that besides the traditional medicine, she had used alternative therapies for years. She kept track of her disease process and how things were progressing. She continued to see her life coach and other supports regularly until close to the end.

Things were uncertain, but she continued to be hopeful and strong both emotionally and psychologically. She took comfort from her support network, which included God, her family, friends, doctors, nurses, personal support workers, and me. We had a good connection, and Carol made sure to call me to keep me updated about anything important related to her condition. It is my belief that both her strong faith and feelings of hopefulness were significant factors that helped her get through the tough days.

Webster's Dictionary defines hope as "a feeling of wanting something to happen and thinking it could happen; a feeling that something good will happen or be true." This was the overriding positive mood that Carol demonstrated that I believe helped to shape her perception of the world, her condition, and her future. From the time I met Carol and throughout her illness her positive attitude, strength of character and resolve were there for all to see. There was a qualitative difference about how she approached people and the world around her. It shaped my perception of her and what I ultimately came to understand about hope. Like many palliative care and end of life patients, Carol had a lot of challenges, but her approach was sure and steady. Eventually, Carol passed away. Her family was very supportive and were with her at the end. I was there to care for and give to Carol but she left me with an enormous gift that was extremely powerful and long lasting.

Throughout my nursing career, I had several other patients with a deep faith in God. I learned how their faith positively affected their journey toward death. It was often a calming force that saw them through the many challenges. For Carol, this was also true. With Carol, I saw a level of hope that I had rarely seen before. It was a prevailing optimism that permeated her being and changed the way everything else seemed to affect her. I felt privileged to get to know her. It was inspiring for me to be part of her journey.

Prison Work
Kirsten's Story

Correctional Nursing

What's it like to be a nurse in a prison? Aren't you scared for your safety? You don't have to see the "really bad ones," do you? Do you know what they are incarcerated for? How can you even provide care to a criminal? The questions are endless when someone finds out that you're an RN in a jail. I graduated from nursing in 2012. In the eight years I've been a nurse, I spent two and a half years working as a correctional nurse. This was my third nursing job. I will forever look back on that time in my nursing career with positive thoughts, and I consider it a great learning experience overall.

Correctional nursing is a little bit of everything all mashed up into one: mental health, obstetrics, acute care, emergency, addiction counsellor, discharge planning… the list goes on. Since correctional nursing is often a side of nursing that is forgotten about, ignored, or even straight-up not known about, I'd like to provide some insight into my experiences while working there and answer some of those "common questions."

FRONT LINE NURSING STORIES

What's It Like to Work in a Prison?

I will always remember the day I pulled into the parking lot of the jail for my job interview. My husband and I had just moved to a new area, so I was looking for a new job. I was super surprised that there was no security to get into the parking lot. I remember looking at the barbed-wire fence around the yard and thinking, *Am I really going to do this?* A jail looks how you would expect it to, inside and out. It took a while for it to become "normal" to me. I was given one shadow day following my interview and job offer to see if it was something I truly wanted to do. It's mainly like working in a hospital, with massively increased security and way less support.

What is Your Role as a Nurse There?

A typical day (from my experience) in the life of a correctional nurse is entering the prison through security, getting reports and being assigned to a unit with 200-plus inmates, preparing for morning med pass, going to the unit, giving out meds, and doing "nurse sick calls," which are things like wound care, blood sugar and blood pressure checks, immunizations, etc. Then documenting, processing orders from the doctors, and preparing for second med pass. During your entire shift, you're on call for all medical emergencies, common ones being overdoses, cardiac issues, and injuries from fights between the inmates. You also frequently do things like suicide screening and alcohol/narcotics withdrawal assessments. There is a medical unit where the sicker inmates go for things like IV meds, peritoneal dialysis, pregnancy checkups, severe wounds, etc. There was also a role for the nurse to do methadone administration. Some days have minimal action; others have more than you feel you can handle. You do a second med pass, report over to night shift, and head out through security to end your day.

Do You Feel Safe?

I never felt safer than when I was working there. All care provided to inmates was done with a correctional officer by your side. As far as I'm concerned, working emergency is far more dangerous. Overall, the inmates are quite respectful of the nurses, and there is a mutual respect (which I guess for a jail setting is like a therapeutic relationship). I only ever felt threatened a couple of times while I was there. Both situations involved me telling an inmate no to their requests for a certain medication. They became upset and said some threatening things that at the time did really upset me. Looking back now, I don't think I'd feel the same. I grew tough skin while working there, but again, overall, it was mainly pleasant or at minimum cordial dealings.

Do You Know What They are Incarcerated For?

Nursing charts did not indicate what charges an inmate was facing. Going into this, I knew it was a maximum-security prison and that there would be every type of crime in there, so to speak. Sometimes the cases were made public in the news, so you knew from that; other times inmates would directly tell you themselves (even though I never asked). I guess I would say maybe fifty percent of the time, you would know what they had done. Honestly, I never cared to know. I saw them all as patients and just dealt with each one the same. I ultimately had a job to do, so the rap list didn't matter.

How did You Ethically Deal with the Job?

As previously stated, patients are patients. As nurses, we deal with all walks of life, and I've dealt with patients "on the outside" who were more terrible to me than most inmates. Just because you're working inside a jail doesn't mean the quality of care you provide can go down. We are obligated as nurses. I'd be lying if I said it wasn't hard at times to look at and deal with people who have done some pretty bad things in their life, but there was also a reward from some who really had just made some poor decisions and were truly good people. You like to think you played a tiny piece in helping to rehabilitate them and always hoped for the best when they were released.

During my time on the job, there was an older inmate who was deemed palliative. Not often as a correctional nurse would you think about providing palliative care, but the situation arose. It ethically tore at me. How do I provide the best end-of-life care to someone who has spent some of their life doing wrong? I really had to work past that situation to see him as my patient and not a dying criminal. What was very interesting to me in this situation was how the other younger inmates cared for this individual in his final days. You see a lot of that in the jail, the young taking care of the old. I think in this situation it gave one particular younger inmate a sense of purpose and a way to give back and try to "right his wrongs." That same younger inmate was a "cleaner," which is an earned and privileged job on the medical unit. I was working one Christmas and we had a big potluck. We made up a plate of our leftovers and gave it to the inmate. He was so happy he cried, and he thanked us for days after. I really saw him that day as a kid who had made some bad decisions, and I felt so sorry for him. Again, being ethically torn and having to take a step back and reflect.

The reality in there is that they are the inmates, and you are the nurse. It doesn't matter if you can relate to them or not. You have a job to do, and being empathic at times can make you weak and at risk in that setting. So imagine everything you've ever been taught about the caring aspect of nursing potentially being a detriment to you in this field. You do really try to see the positive in them, and it was very disappointing when he [the cleaner] was released clean and sober and ready to take on the world, and came back days later after paramedics and police found him in a laundromat, passed out with a needle still in his arm. That was a frustrating part of the job, and it opened my eyes to the nasty world of addiction.

What's different about correctional nursing?

Safety is always first. Nursing tasks do not get done if the safety of yourself, correctional officers, or other inmates is at risk. You have to learn the lingo. There are so many slang terms that you have to get used to and even use in some circumstances. You are always being watched and followed. You constantly must think about the dangers of the job, like you can never leave a pen or even a paper clip sitting out. Your body is always facing the exit. Keys are secured to you, and no cellphones are allowed in the facility. You don't have access to most hospital equipment, and a lot of inmates end up going to hospital for further assessment due to lack of supports in the prison.

What are Some of the Craziest Things You've Seen?

I went to do a nurse sick call one day. The inmate I was seeing was a new transfer in from another jail, so I hadn't seen his chart yet. The request just said, "wound care." When he came into the room, he had a bandage wrapped around his head. I asked what was going on under there. He responded, "Someone bit my ear off." I laughed, thinking he was joking, and he said, "No, seriously, miss" (they always refer to the nurses as "miss"). I took the bandage off to see a large chunk at the top of his ear was necrotic. He wasn't lying. Another inmate had attempted to bite his ear off in an altercation at his previous jail, and the attempt to repair it had failed. I was blown away that someone would do that, but after working there for some time, I saw all kinds of altercation wounds, from straight-up broken knuckles to completely unconscious head traumas. Thankfully, I was never working during a riot or inmate suicide, which have both happened to most of my fellow co-workers there and, of course, are very traumatic situations.

I was also always surprised by the level of artwork in their jail tattoos. Inmates are very resourceful and would literally make their own tattoo kits and tattoo other inmates. Inevitably, the nurse would end up seeing them for infected wounds shortly after. I can still to this day pick out a jail tattoo.

All in all, it was one of my favourite jobs. I take pride in being able to be tough and get the job done in a vastly different setting. Who knows where the road will lead? I would never say never to going back to work in the correctional system. That's the great joy in nursing. It can take you down all kinds of paths, including those in lockdown.

FRONT LINE NURSING STORIES

A Remote Visit in the North Bay Area
Carol's Story

When I was working in North Bay and the surrounding areas, we had lots of very remote patients who we could only get to by boat or snowmobile. There was one person I had to see who you could drive to in the summer. Sometimes you could drive there in the spring or fall, depending on the weather and if it wasn't too wet. The patient lived through miles of marshland in a remote area that had a track built up with fill. The drive was meant more for a four-wheeler than a truck. It was an iffy drive unless the road was dry. If you could not drive because it was raining, or if it was winter, the patient would come out to get you on his snowmobile.

One day, because of the weather, the patient came to pick me up to do my home visit. I drove in with him on his snowmobile. I did the visit. It was a beautiful day. The snow was packed down, so I decided I would just walk back.

I was walking down the track and was about halfway there. It was getting colder and colder. I thought maybe it wasn't such a good idea after all. My briefcase was getting heavier and heavier. I changed my mind and turned around to walk back.

There in my steps were these giant moose tracks. When I turned around there was no moose visible, but the tracks were right on top of my footprints. The moose had been walking behind me the whole time. I didn't realize because I was probably making a lot of noise clomping along the track. I was busy thinking about my next visit and not paying attention to my surroundings. I was engrossed in my own thoughts. I was out of sight of the house and had to pass some trees. The moose didn't come back out from behind the trees. I couldn't move very fast, but I hustled back to the house as quickly as possible.

You hear some wild moose stories in that area. This includes moose attacking cars when they are in a bad mood or in season.

At that time, we did not carry cellphones. We had bag phones that you plugged into your car lighter. A lot of the offices in the small towns didn't have three-pronged plugs. They had knob and tubing wiring. If you had problems using your computer for assessments, then you had to pull out your paper copy. This would have been around 2003, when we started the computer assessment. Before computer assessment, each case manager had a paper assessment. On the paper form, you had a broad outline with headings: Medical Status, Physical Status, Emotional, Social Support, etc. You asked your own questions, gathered the information, and completed the service plan, which included the goals of care. These were all completed in conjunction with the patient and family. Consent was always obtained. From your assessment, you figured out what the areas of strength and weakness were and then determined the needs and services required. It was a much simpler time. We did it, and I think we did it well. We made good eye contact and made some very good connections.

I experienced many challenges while working out in those remote areas. I went to homes with tons of cats. Some homes had chickens walking around in the house. On occasion, I had to work surrounded by cockroaches. And, of course, it was not unusual for me to visit homes where there was manure on the floor. The manure would be there because sometimes on a farm they track the stuff from the yard and barn into the home and it gets walked over and into parts of the house. Initially, it might be quite a surprise. You would go for your visit, get shocked, get over it, and find a way to meet their needs. The police are familiar with the social problems in the different areas. As a health care provider, you are usually not going to change their world, so you do what you can and leave.

Reflections on Teaching and Learning
Marian's Story

I was teaching nursing at a community college, which had gone to a four-year degree program. In this program, students spent two years at the college and then two more years studying at university. The schools had a cooperative agreement.

Teaching nursing was a great experience for me. I learned about the curriculum and about student learning. Getting into teaching was an easy transition for me as I had previously been involved in adult education. I taught expectant parents the stages of labour and delivery and what they should expect as they progressed toward the delivery of their babies. I taught a course on documentation to nurses. I supervised practicums with personal support workers, and I had several other teaching experiences. These were mostly with adult learners. In contrast, the students at the college were mostly new graduates from high school.

The nursing course I taught consisted of both a theoretical component and a practical component. I was teaching the theoretical component. The philosophy of the college was cooperative learning. Collaboration, communication, and group work were seen as important aspects of the course and teaching. Group work involved learning within the classroom setting and outside the classroom with group project work. Part of my job was to evaluate and provide a grade on team function and process.

"Reflective progress notes" were used in the practical setting, but they were used when needed in the classroom as well. Writing a reflective progress note was a way for students to look at a situation and analyze it to determine how it could have been handled more effectively. Reflection provided an opportunity for students to examine their thoughts, feelings, and behaviour in a situation.

Classroom rules were discussed and agreed upon by myself and the students at the outset of each course I was teaching. Mutual respect was deemed to be essential. In this environment, I had many wonderful encounters with students. There were also a few encounters that were more challenging. I will share with you one of the more challenging ones, as I think it will demonstrate the value of using the reflective practice approach.

I had a student who I will call Victor. He had been a student in the three-year Registered Nursing (RN) Program but had dropped out for personal reasons. He returned to college after some time and was enrolled in the degree program. That is when I met him.

In class, Victor did not look happy, although he did participate in class group work. He never smiled and always seemed tense. He had a negative vibe about him. I would even call it a "chip on his shoulder."

There were times when students worked together on games that would bring forth parts of the learning they needed to do. On this one day, we had just finished the group work and I proceeded to do some lecturing. There were two students talking loudly. One of them was Victor. Their voices were obviously a disruption to me and the other students. I asked them to please refrain from talking as it was disrupting the class. One student stopped talking and apologized. Victor became irritated, breathed out a long, loud sigh, rolled his eyes, and defiantly folded his arms. He was very irritated. He wasn't pleased with the request, and his non-verbal communication demonstrated this. I requested that he leave the class and speak to the faculty coordinator before returning. He refused to leave and said he would remain quiet.

He attended the community portion of the class the same afternoon. He had not seen the coordinator or made an appointment as I had requested.

Two weeks before this occurrence, I had asked Victor to complete a reflective progress note. I requested this because I thought he needed to reflect on his communication and attitude during the class. It was significant enough that it needed to be addressed. A few students had approached me and let me know they were unsettled by Victor's attitude toward me and that it was affecting them and the learning environment. He was also distant from classmates. As they saw his behaviour escalate, they seemed to move away from him.

At the end of class, I asked Victor to stay as I wanted to talk with him. I requested a copy of his reflective note that had been assigned two weeks earlier. He told me he had not yet completed it. His attitude was sarcastic. I told him I had made an appointment for him to follow up with the coordinator later that afternoon. He said he was unable to make it. I requested that he cancel the appointment and reschedule as soon as possible.

There were several graded assignments as part of the course. The class had handed in their essays, and I had read and marked them. At the next class, I planned to hand back their essays at the end of class. When I started the class, Victor asked for his essay results. He did not want to wait until the end of class to get them. He was agitated and upset that he had to wait for his results. We took a mid-morning break. Some students went outside, and I went to the washroom.

When I returned, I was informed by another student that Victor had gone into my bag where I had my laptop. He was looking to find his mark on his paper. The list of students and their marks were all in the file. I could hardly believe it. I felt that Victor had not only violated me but had been in a position to look at other students' marks and essays, which I considered confidential. None of this was okay.

I did my best to remain objective and to discuss things with him. I kept the faculty coordinator updated, and she did the same with me. Victor was anxious and said he was not even aware of his negative communication in the beginning. Eventually, Victor acknowledged that he had a lot going on in his personal life and that he had lost control of himself. Victor needed to correct his communication and adjust the path he was headed down. Several reflective progress notes and a collaborative plan were used to help Victor and the process along. By writing about his thoughts and feelings, Victor was able to understand his motivations and to identify what he had done wrong. He developed insight into his own behaviour. He acknowledged that his relationship with other students was affected by his attitude. He told me he was genuinely upset with himself for his behaviours. Basically, Victor took responsibility for his actions and decided that he would change his ways going forward. I believed him.

I did not have another course with Victor once this course was over, but I do believe he was different. I saw how he was so much better in my class and how his progress notes reflected his desire to change. Years later, I met up with him when our paths crossed briefly. He was working as a nurse. He seemed settled and professional.

A situation like this would have been handled quite differently when I trained to become an RN. At that time, discipline and compliance to instructions were required. A student who demonstrated defiant behaviour would have been either expelled from the program, put on probation, and/or minimally received a reprimand. There would have been little consideration for the reasons why such behaviour had occurred. Victor's behaviour was, of course, inappropriate, but with good guidance, he ultimately improved his approach to problem solving.

When I was teaching, I learned the value of having a supportive dean and faculty. They were calm, confident, and had a lot of experience to draw from. Their communication skills were good. I felt valued and supported. I felt they trusted me. I learned that nursing faculty deal with so much. It is not just about preparing for class, delivering the content, and marking the exams and copious submissions about the many aspects of nursing. The professors can be a big support to students as they experience academic and personal challenges through their student journey. I learned to appreciate the hard work and energy required to help get a student either on track or back on track. I realized the amount of work the professors put in to get the job done both academically and otherwise.

9. Art Meets Science

The foundation of nursing is science. During their education, nurses study concepts and theories related to nursing which provide principles that underpin practice. Areas of study include but are not limited to: anatomy and physiology, growth and development, pharmacology, pathophysiology, systems theory and courses in the social sciences. Nurses study specialty areas of paediatrics, obstetrics, mental health and community health. Practicums in different areas serve to enhance and integrate the knowledge bases. Nurses rely on general and scientific knowledge from many disciplines. The combination of this knowledge is the starting point for the practice of nursing. Knowledge of physical, psychological, and social characteristics help direct a nurse's assessment and intervention with patients and families.

The art of nursing goes beyond the scientific knowledge and includes knowledge that is non-scientific—specifically, knowledge of the patient's experience. This knowledge is subjective, as it originates in part from the relationship between the nurse and patient. It includes knowledge about the patient's feelings, thoughts about illness, and values and goals. Who is this patient and what are the patient's strengths and limitations? What are this patient's needs and what will facilitate growth or transition? By understanding these, the nurse can gather the pieces of information and understand the patient, who is always more than the sum of their parts. Each person is unique. The art of nursing is demonstrated when the nurse understands the gestalt of the situation and responds in a way that meets the needs of the patient in the moment. Intuition often comes into play.

The stories in this chapter show how nurses practice the art of nursing as they effectively deal with specific patients (and families), their medical situations, needs, and movements through their trajectory of illness and the healing process. Artful encounters can be as brief and simple as a look, a gesture, words, or active listening. Examples of these have been pointed out throughout the book. They can also be more complex, the journey through the birthing process or transition toward a peaceful death. I have chosen the following stories to illustrate how nursing comes alive as an art form and how it can play a pivotal role in the healing process.

What Was Not Said
Sharon M.'s Story

Before I graduated with my diploma in nursing, one of my professors encouraged us all to subscribe to at least two nursing journals during our careers. After graduation, I took that to heart and subscribed to *Journal of Emergency Nursing* (JEN), a journal of research, statistics, and best practices. The other journal I chose was *Nursing*, which was more hands-on and provided more practical information. The last page usually featured a nurse's experience with a patient. I remember there was one story about an ICU nurse caring for an intubated patient. She spoke with him every day to explain to him the procedure that was being utilized. She also talked about other things. She told him the date, time, and what the weather was like.

When the RN was on maternity leave, the patient recovered. He returned sometime later to the unit in order to thank the nurses and ICU staff. He was looking to thank that one nurse who spoke with him whenever she was assigned to his care. He did not know her name. He then heard her voice in the background and knew it was her. I carried that story with me throughout my nursing career.

One shift, when I was working in ER, a teen was admitted to our trauma unit after a car accident. Unfortunately, death was certain. I was the main nurse for this patient. I was also a strong advocate for not tidying up the room too much until the patient/family were gone. The MD and I went into the "Quiet Room" and informed the parents that their son had died. I stayed with the family. I inquired if they wanted to see their son. I prepared them for the chaotic appearance of the room.

Once in the room where their son was laid out, his body still warm, the parents were beside themselves. Both were expressing feelings of guilt, especially the mom. She felt she should not have hurried him. She was also upset because she hadn't said "I love you."

I then asked the parents if they wanted to hug their son. If they did, I would need some help lifting him. The mother was overcome with hurt and guilt. I encouraged her to speak to her son and tell him whatever she meant to say before he left home. No one knew if he could hear. Might it be that his spirit was still nearby? It was so difficult.

Later that month, I received a note from the hospital foundation. The parents had donated money in my name for the care that their son and family had received.

Some Tricks of the Trade
Sharon M.'s Story

In this next story, Sharon shares some of the "tricks of the trade" she has acquired over many years of practice working with kids. She has an ability to assess the kids and make good judgments. In this story she demonstrates how the art of nursing comes alive as she takes her care to another level.

As a diploma nurse, I worked for years before returning to university to get my BScN. I worked predominately in pediatric emergency departments, as well as a year in adult ICU. I gained a lot of amazing experience. There was one day in the emergency department that stands out.

A child with spina bifida arrived in the ER post-operatively. He had received corrective surgery with the insertion of a Harrington rod and been discharged home. Sometime after discharge, he arrived back at our hospital. He had spent the night in our ER with the complaint of "spitting up." Due to staff shortage, I arrived on days and was met by the usual chaotic backlog of patients. I assessed this child. His vital signs where not within normal range. He had a distended abdomen. The pediatrician on that shift trusted the nurses' judgment. I assessed the child and spoke with the physician, who agreed that the child should have a nasogastric tube (N/G) inserted and connected to low pressure. I measured and marked the abdomen, inserted the N/G. I have forgotten now how many litres were drained, but I remember that it was an incredible amount. I cleaned out the child's mouth with a lemon glycerin stick. I washed him and applied cream over his body, changed his gown and bedsheets, and found a warm blanket and some pillows to help position him more comfortably. I did what I call "basic nursing care." It was one of my most rewarding shifts. His vitals dropped within normal range and he was so much more comfortable.

I think sometimes as nurses we focus on the many advances in tasks that nurses do, such as starting IVs, drawing blood, listening to chests on asthmatics, and starting Ventolin as a standard order. Over my forty years of practice, nursing has come a long way. I look back at that one shift, knowing that my college professors would be so proud of my basic nursing care and my advocacy for a child without a voice.

The art of nursing is sometimes difficult to articulate. Sometimes kids are petrified of nurses. This is especially true when parents wrongly inform them that nurses "give needles if they misbehave"! This type of messaging is one of my pet peeves. Over time, I tried to come up with some reassuring phrases. Having blood pressure taken can be very frightening for children. With boys I would say, "I just need to find out if you have really strong muscles." After taking the pressure, I would say, "WOW, you are really strong." With girls (I know I am being sexist, but it worked) I would say, "I am going to give your arm a bit of a hug." It felt good when I started to hear EMS using that phrase! WOW!

Something I learned from my professors in my diploma course was to taste the medications that are being given. A mom trying to give her child some erythromycin—godawful stuff—could not get her son to take it. I asked her to taste it. She gave me the dirtiest look afterward. It made sense to me. How can you give something to a child if you don't know how it tastes? I was always honest with kids and would tell them it tasted "yucky." So I would offer the kid a Popsicle to numb the taste. I would tell the child to swallow the yucky medicine and then take another bite of the Popsicle. It helped and accomplished the task.

Sarcoma and Palliation
Louise's Story

Janet was a young adult when I first met her. She lived with her boyfriend in a townhouse. She had been diagnosed with right shoulder sarcoma and was on chemotherapy with the hope that this tumour would shrink enough to allow surgery to take place. She had been sent home with a PICC line in place being used as a direct access point for chemotherapy. The nurses in the hospital could administer the chemo medication using the PICC line without having to puncture her veins each time treatment was scheduled.

Janet had been referred to our agency by a Toronto hospital where her chemotherapy was taking place. Her needs were assessed there, with a request for in-home nursing between her scheduled visits to Toronto for chemotherapy. The role of the in-home nurses was to manage the site of the PICC, monitor for signs and symptoms of deterioration, and provide support for pain management. Janet required regular dressing care around the insertion site of the PICC and flushing of the device.

She had not been on our program long before her mother called our agency in distress. She said that each trip to and from Toronto was getting more and more difficult. Her pain was not well controlled. Every movement was difficult. When she was first admitted to our service, she could get out of bed and go to the bathroom to do her own shower. She could use the toilet in her home. But within days, she went from being independent to totally dependent. She could no longer get out of bed or walk on her own. Her condition was getting worse and she could no longer travel by car to Toronto.

As an interim measure, the case manager on our support team who took the call arranged for an ambulance to transport Janet to Toronto for her treatment. She requested that a hospital bed be put in her home and that an occupational therapist do an assessment for additional equipment in the home. There was a request for an urgent home visit, and her file was transferred to me. I spoke with her mom on the phone to book the home visit. Janet had given us permission to talk with her mom and to have her on the contact list. Although she didn't live with her daughter, mom was her main support and spent long hours at her home looking after her.

It was the middle of winter, and the steps up to the front door were slippery and dangerous. Janet's mother greeted me at the front door. She was calm and looked very concerned. Behind her was Janet's partner Tom, who was a big guy, around six feet tall. He was twenty-four years old but looked much younger. They welcomed me with few words. I was ushered to the back bedroom of the home, where Janet was sitting upright in the hospital bed. Janet was a tiny slip of a thing with short blond hair.

There was an invisible circle of tension around the right side of Janet's body. I soon learned that it radiated around her right shoulder and arm. I realized that the imaginary lines of protection were there so she could ensure nothing would touch this painful part of her body. There was a radius of about eight to ten inches surrounding her limb that was untouchable. Every look on her face and every movement or lack thereof was proof of the pain and protection of this extremity. My focus was on her protected area and I noted that this limb was at least twice the size of her other arm. Her fingers on that side were very swollen. She was frozen in one position and frightened to death to move at all. She refused to turn on either side. Her arm was in a sling and her hand dangled out of it. Her left hand held the right one up.

At the time of my first visit, both Janet's mom and Tom stayed with me while I talked with her. I could tell she was getting tired. The remainder of my visit was spent with mom in the living room while Tom stayed in the bedroom with Janet.

Janet's mom was an amazing woman. She was open and honest with me and gave me a lot of information. She reported that a biopsy had been done on Janet's shoulder and confirmed it was sarcoma. Within six months, it had spread to both lungs. She was hopeful that they would be able to contain the sarcoma and then do the surgery.

She told me how Janet and Tom had only been together for a couple of years. They both worked and they were able to support themselves independently in the townhouse. Tom did physical labour; he worked in the construction industry which required heavy lifting. Janet worked in the tech industry.

Mom told me how Tom was overwhelmed and had difficulty managing Janet's care. He did spend as much time with her as possible and did a lot of the cooking. He emptied the bedpan but had a lot of trouble taking care of the basin contents after Janet defecated. He wanted to be there for Janet but was finding it very stressful. Mom told me that Tom didn't really understand the seriousness of her condition or what her needs were. In a short period, Janet had gone from taking care of herself to needing help to transfer in and out of bed and on and off the toilet. Whenever she moved from the bed to the commode for toileting, the pain in her shoulder and arm was excruciating. She needed help with transfers and to wipe herself.

Her condition had not only deteriorated, but her pain was also not controlled. She had a pain specialist and oncologist in Toronto. This was about a ninety-minute drive from where Janet lived. The doctors were not able to do home visits. Mom spoke with them on the phone regularly. The in-home nurses provided support and guidance for her. Mom was the one who gave the subcutaneous medication. She also poured Janet's pills and made sure they were properly administered. She went home each day to spend time with her spouse and other family members but returned to Janet and stayed late into the evening.

Janet's family doctor wasn't well-versed in palliative care, including pain management. This was the main area of concern at the time of my visit. Janet's body was tense and frozen, as the slightest movement sent shock waves down her shoulder and arm.

After completing my interview with Janet, her mother and Tom and then alone with mom, I felt I had a very good idea of the home situation and Janet's condition. Prior to the visit, I had spoken with the primary nurse, and together we acknowledged the need for better medical follow-up and palliative care in the home setting. We agreed that given Janet's challenge with pain control, it would be best for her to have a physician in the area who was an expert dealing with people like her. Although the Toronto physicians were caring and competent, it was difficult for them to administer day-to-day care from afar without seeing Janet regularly. I spoke with mom about the importance of having a physician close by who could do home visits, assess pain, and work closely with the in-home nurses. Mom agreed for me to call the family physician and have a conversation about this with him. I encouraged her to do the same.

Through my conversation with mom, I realized that she was expecting Janet to get better. She was hoping that the experimental chemotherapy treatment would work so she could have the surgery and improve. I knew from the information I had and my past experiences that the most we could hope for was good pain management, palliative care in the home, and quality of life for Janet while she stayed home. According to mom, no one in Toronto had spoken to her about palliative care. I knew it was vital that she understood the situation so she could support Janet through her deterioration. My other concern was that Janet, her family, her partner, the nurses, and I would need the support of a good palliative physician. We needed to work as a team for Janet's sake. We needed someone to do home visits and someone to liaise with the Toronto physicians and take accountability for Janet's pain control in the community.

Janet's mom and I spoke at length about things. I was careful with the words I used. I tried to be sensitive, but what sensitive words are there to convey to someone that their daughter, a person they adored, was going to need all the support they could get as she approached death? I did this one step at a time and one interaction at a time. I didn't tell her directly that she was going to die, but I could see that she was starting to understand. She was very slowly but undeniably making mental notes of things. She allowed herself to start to make connections. She came to understand that her daughter would need the full complement of professionals—including a palliative care physician—so her needs would be met in a timely manner and she would be spared as much pain as possible.

This was a difficult visit, but one that I am happy I made. The issues were discussed, and now there was a plan to address some of the more pressing problems. I encouraged mom to call me if needed. She agreed, and after that day she called me regularly.

When I left the home that day, I believe Janet's mom knew that I cared about all of them and that I meant well. We made a connection. I felt that she knew she could call me any time. I knew that the first barrier of defense was penetrated, and that mom would slowly allow herself to understand. Our goal when I left was to find out from the family doctor if he was willing and able to care for Janet at home. If not, would he agree to have a specialist in the community fulfill this role? The primary nurse and I had already decided on the physician we thought would be best able to care for Janet if the family doctor was unable to do so.

The family doctor wasn't comfortable managing Janet's pain and was transparent about his limited experience with palliative care. He agreed to our choice of visiting physician. I made the call to the palliative care doctor, who agreed to take on Janet's care. She needed to be sure the physicians in Toronto were all right with this plan. This type of thing could be sensitive, and it was prudent for us, as nurses and case manager, to be careful not to step on anyone's toes. Our chosen physician made the calls to Toronto and spoke with the physicians there. Everyone was now on the same page and we could proceed in a more case-coordinated and effective manner.

Mom did call me when needed. I spoke often with the primary nurse. At one point, mom was quite concerned as Janet needed complete care and Tom wasn't providing help with sponge bathing. Janet was at great risk for skin breakdown. She stayed in the same position most of the day and refused to move onto either side or into any position other than sitting up. I made another home visit to try to get Tom to agree to have a personal support worker come in to help, but he did not want anyone else doing Janet's care. He told me that everything was "under control." It was a delicate situation: Mom could see that her basic needs were not being adequately met but felt helpless as Tom could not admit this. I had the nurses review the skin care, positioning, and transfers education with both Tom and mom. We got a pressure-relieving device for the hospital bed. Janet was sensitive to her partner's feelings, and mom did not want to create any more stress than there needed to be. She was also worried about her daughter's care. This intervention helped, but there continued to be issues on and off over the next several weeks.

The occupational therapist made suggestions for devices and equipment to facilitate Janet's function. The local palliative care physician was able to get Janet's pain under control and provide in-home visits and support. The primary nurse kept in regular contact with me, so together we could work as a team to ensure Janet and the family's needs were met.

I went on vacation. Every so often, my thoughts would wander and I would think about Janet and her family. I wondered how they were doing and if Janet was still alive.

When I got back, I had a message from Janet's mom, requesting that I call her. While I was away, Janet had gone to our local hospice. She was only there a few days before she passed away. I spoke with one of the staff members at hospice to see how things had gone there. While Janet was slipping slowly into death, Tom was still asking when she was going to get better and be able to come home. These questions were being asked twenty-four to forty-eight hours before she died.

I never made it to the funeral. By the time I was able to connect with mom, it was too late. I only met Janet, her mother, and Tom a few times. I spoke with mom a lot on the phone. I believe that I was able to establish a trusting relationship and provided the coordinated help for the family on their very difficult journey. I will always remember Janet, her mom, and Tom. We worked as a team. The open, honest communication between Janet, her family, the nurses, physician, and myself allowed this transition to happen in a way that made me feel comfortable and satisfied with the outcome.

FRONT LINE NURSING STORIES

Integrating Art and Science
Amy's Story

A nursing story that has always stood out for me was the summer I took my first nursing job as a student at a Victorian Order of Nurses Alzheimer's day centre. I was part of a team that worked with adults living with cognitive decline, dementia, and Alzheimer's. This program allowed family members, spouses, and adult children to receive some respite or support for their loved one. My role was to spend time with the patients, keep them focused on a variety of activities, go for a walk, and help them take part in activities that they used to enjoy (e.g., gardening, baking, physical activity). Really just be with them in whatever moment they were in.

There was a particular patient who they often paired me with. He responded well to me. I found his personal story made a strong impression on me. He was in his seventies and had been diagnosed with Alzheimer's. In his working life, he had been a successful CEO and entrepreneur. He had been a thought leader in his time. Here I was, observing and seeing the effects that this disease had on his movements, on his thinking, and his behaviour, on him, on his family. One moment he could be lucid, and then the next moment, you could watch him lose his cognitive thought or the words to express himself. It was heartbreaking. He was frustrated at times. Emotional. I felt for him and his family.

Compassion and caring were at the root of how I was understood as a student and, interestingly, how I sought to see my patients and their families throughout my nursing career. When I reflect now, the art and science of nursing have always been a part of who I am, which blend of science and the art of caring for and working with people. Assessing and seeking to understand and care for the human body, appreciating how disease affects normal functioning, and taking into consideration so many factors. But, most importantly, considering the individual who lives within. The more I reflect, the more I appreciate the many complexities that can impact one's health and wellness along the lifespan, and I also appreciate the valuable role a compassionate and caring nurse can play in supporting patients along their journey.

Amyotrophic Lateral Sclerosis (ALS)

Amyotrophic lateral sclerosis (ALS), otherwise known as Lou Gehrig's disease, is a motor neuron disease that causes death of the neurons controlling voluntary muscles. ALS can start as a muscle weakness or twitching that gradually gets worse. It often begins with weakness of the arms or legs, or difficulty speaking or swallowing. It can also include mild difficulty with thinking. Most people have pain. A person with ALS eventually loses the ability to walk, use their hands, speak, swallow. and breathe.

The patients in the next two stories both had a diagnosis of ALS, but they were very different people, with different values, needs, expectations, stages of life, coping skills, and families. The trajectory of the illnesses was different. The two scenarios show the uniqueness of each patient and family and their needs. Consequently, interventions and responses provided by the nurse facilitated desired outcomes for each patient and family.

Scenario One: A Couple in Extreme Distress
Margaret's Story

I was a case manager working in the community in eastern Ontario. I had been called into the manager's office. She wanted to transfer a complex and dissatisfied couple to my caseload. I called the patient's husband George to introduce myself. It became apparent that his upset and frustration was related mainly to the service of the personal support workers (PSWs), what they had not done or had not done right. I decided to do a home visit the next day. George's wife was a palliative care patient.

This couple was interesting. They were socially and physically very active. George was a retired professional and well-educated. Sandra, his wife, was in her mid to late fifties. She too was well-educated and retired.

FRONT LINE NURSING STORIES

The couple was very active and fit. They were part of a group that ran daily. A few months earlier, Sandra had been out running as per her regular routine but was no longer able to keep pace with the group. She had repeated weakness in her foot. This was an early sign that something was wrong. Her mobility continued to deteriorate. She saw her family physician and from there was referred to a specialist for consultation. She was diagnosed with ALS.

When I did the home visit, the couple let me know about some of the issues related to the home care they were receiving. For the most part, according to the couple, the nurses were doing all right. Much of their stress centred around the PSW assistance. They did not think the PSWs were doing well with transfers, bathing, or feeding. There was not the continuity they expected from the providers. George felt he had gone over this issue time and again with the PSW supervisor, to no avail. There was a generalized deep tension in the room.

I suggested we have a conference in the home and include the providers. The couple was not only agreeable but welcomed this idea. During my time with them, I concluded that George was very anxious. He did not know what to expect. This was a man who was used to having control over things, but in this case, he had very little control and was extremely frustrated. This frustration was exhibited in his anger. I think he felt that he was not being heard and that he was also frightened of the entire situation. Sandra, on the other hand, was anxious about this new diagnosis. She had been reading up on her illness and was overwhelmed.

The day of the conference, I bumped into the PSW supervisor on the driveway before we entered the home. She was relatively new to her role with the agency. I gave her a heads-up about what George had told me were some of his issues related to the patient's care. I wanted her to be ready for what he might say. I was surprised when she minimized the issues of lack of continuity of providers and her disregard for how the couple wanted things done. I did not expect her attitude. In my previous encounters with other supervisors, they seemed more than willing to work as a team. This person's attitude was different. I concluded that it might be part of the problem. I reminded the supervisor that the agency's expectation was to develop mutual goals, with the patient and family participating in the problem-solving process. We wanted a high quality of care, we wanted the patient and family to be satisfied, and we all needed to play our part to achieve this. That included her, too.

The conference was held at the home with the patient, her husband, the nurse, the palliative care physician, the PSW supervisor, and me. We cooperatively developed an agenda. There was discussion about the main complaint, which concerned the PSW support. George spoke about a lack of continuity and a lack of detail about how things were done. He spoke about some issues related to individual competence. Although George needed respite himself, he did not feel that he could leave his wife alone in the home with the PSW while he went out.

Talking openly about the issues helped the couple feel they had some say in their care. Opinions were shared. George started to feel he had some control over his life and the care provided to his wife. Changes were made to service delivery.

Over time, the PSW issues improved. It was decided that the supervisor would draw up a schedule that indicated which PSW would be coming when. Some of the procedures, such as transfers for bathing, were written out so that all PSWs would do them the same way and lessen the anxiety felt by Sandra. The couple requested that the supervisor come to the home and do some hands-on teaching with the agency staff when needed. Sandra liked routine, and it was a small price to pay to ensure she was comfortable with her care.

We had a few more conferences in the home over the duration of her illness. I believe this helped the couple sort out issues of concern and gave them a feeling of safety, security and control.

As time went on, Sandra began having difficulty swallowing. A dietician was added for nutritional reasons. As Sandra's condition worsened, she could no longer speak in such a way that she could be understood. We had a speech and language therapist involved who developed an effective communication system for Sandra. This worked for everyone and certainly lessened the extreme anxiety that Sandra was feeling. There was a respiratory therapist involved as well. At some point a BiPAP machine, a positive-pressure ventilator, was set up in the home. The do-not-resuscitate (DNR) order was addressed by the physician. Sandra and her spouse wanted the death to be at home, so an Expected Death in the Home (EDITH) protocol and chart were set up. There was also a communication chart for all providers to use. All service providers could record and share important data here, and it was expected they would keep the file up to date so each provider knew what the others were doing.

As Sandra's condition deteriorated, the nurses visited more often to ensure that she was comfortable. The patient received general nursing care, medication, suctioning, and ventilation care. Respite care was provided for George. The community agency where I worked had limits to what could be provided, but the couple received all that they needed within the specified boundaries. The physician visited whenever it was deemed necessary and provided education about the trajectory of the disease and support throughout the decline. George also remained involved throughout. He got some needed respite and was reminded to call me whenever he felt he needed to do so. It was a team effort. When I visited the patient, I noticed that the level of stress in the home was reduced and manageable.

A short time after Sandra's passing, I received a card at our agency. It was sent to me to thank the people involved in Sandra's care for the support provided to her and the family. It especially wanted to thank the nurses who worked at the bedside with Sandra. I sent a copy to the nursing agency so they could share this with their dedicated nurses. A copy was sent to the PSW agency so the staff there could be thanked as well.

In this case, it was important to recognize the complexity of the situation. The couple's needs and expectations were important to recognize and acknowledge. Their anxiety level was high. They needed a lot of reassurance, education, and support to come to terms with what was happening. The couple needed to feel they had some control over the care. They knew they did not have control over the eventual outcome.

MARIAN FACCIOLO

Scenario Two: Sisters Needing Support
Margaret's Story

We received a referral from the ALS clinic for an elderly lady living in our catchment area. I reviewed the information. The patient, Faith, had just been diagnosed with ALS and was declining rapidly. The ALS clinic had made a notation that it was questioning palliative care for her.

Our agency received the referral on a Friday. I called to set up a visit for the following Monday afternoon.

Faith was in her late eighties. She lived with her sister in a rural area outside the city limits. It was snowing and the roads were slick on the day I drove out to meet them. Her sister had given me good directions, so I found the home without difficulty, parked the car at the roadside, and trudged through the snow to the front door. As I approached, I wondered what this visit would bring on this snowy day. What surprises would I find behind that door and what kind of people would I meet today?

The front door opened, and I was greeted by an elderly lady who was neatly dressed. She seemed a little tentative, as this was all new to her. We exchanged introductions and Maureen, the patient's sister, ushered me into the living room, where the visiting nurse was finishing up her assessment.

The nurse was a bit flustered. The suction machine was in a box on the floor. It had been sent out at our agency's request and had arrived at the home that morning. The nurse was planning to teach Maureen how to use it, but she was unable to do so because the company had sent the wrong equipment. The machine and the tubing did not go together. The nurse had already called the equipment company and requested that a new machine be sent out as soon as possible. The company agreed to send a new one early the next morning, so the nurse planned to visit the next day to do the teaching. A nursing visit frequency was established.

I introduced myself to Faith. She was sitting on the couch and looked tired and pale. She was frail, short of breath, and unable to talk. After Faith was diagnosed with "ALS …deteriorating," the clinic had requested she have a nurse to teach suctioning; a speech language pathologist (SLP) for speech difficulties, communication, and choking risk; and a dietician to address choking spells in conjunction with the SLP, assess oral intake, and develop a regime to counter the weight loss and to make recommendations about food intake. I had been asked to visit to do an overall assessment, establish a plan of care, and look at her personal care needs.

Maureen was her main caregiver and, to this point, was helping with personal care, meal preparation, dressing, transfers, and supervision with ambulation for short distances. This patient and her sister had very little informal support. There was only a distant relative in the area, and a brother who lived out of the country for six months of the year. He was not in the country while all this was happening.

I could see right away that Maureen needed help to manage her sister's care in the home. I set up to do the interview in the living room. Faith was involved as much as she could be, given her speech issues. She did try to speak but all that came out were sounds. I could not understand what she was trying to communicate. She was given paper and a pen to write things down. Her sister was a great support and provided the information needed to conduct the assessment. Faith listened intently.

Faith had been living with her sister for a couple of years. She had sold her home and moved in with Maureen. It was just the two of them living there. One could easily see that there was a strong bond between them. They had quiet but effective non-verbal communication. Most of the time, they didn't even need to look at each other, as Maureen answered the questions with ease and provided the information. Most of the time, Faith simply looked on. She was very alert and oriented. She had all her faculties and she trusted her sister with her life. At times, Faith would answer and Maureen would translate. Maureen understood, while I could not decipher what Faith was saying.

Faith had been to see her family doctor about a year before with various complaints. Tests were done, but they were not certain what was wrong. She was having trouble with swallowing and had a lot of saliva buildup. A referral was made to the ALS clinic and specialists for consultation. They had seen her just a week earlier, and that is where we came in. Apparently, it is unusual for someone of Faith's age to get ALS, but it can happen. She had lost a lot of weight over three months and was quite frail. She was only able to walk a short distance with her walker from her room to the living room. She was short of breath with any exertion. Trying to talk exhausted her more.

I completed the assessment and documented everything on the computer. The referral source had questioned whether she was palliative, but I wasn't sure why they would question this. It was clear to me that Faith was palliative and most likely approaching the end of her life.

Near the end of the interview, Faith was trying desperately to communicate directly with me. No matter how hard I tried, I could not understand her words. Her sister said, "She is saying that she wants to die at home." I nodded that I understood. I told Maureen that it was important to get a family doctor in the area. Faith's family physician was located too far away. We needed someone who could do home visits and support Faith, Maureen, the nurses, and other providers in the home setting. When Maureen agreed, I told her I would work on this and get a physician in place for her.

I left the room with Maureen for a short period so she could show me the bathroom and bedroom setup. This way, I could determine what other equipment might be needed to facilitate Faith's care at home. During our walk to the other rooms, I mentioned to Maureen that it was very important to have a do-not-resuscitate (DNR) order in place. I explained that without this, health care providers, including ambulance attendants and paramedics, would be obliged to do resuscitation if Faith stopped breathing. Maureen agreed but requested that this not be discussed with Faith until the following day. She said she did understand the importance of this.

Faith was short of breath. I asked about oxygen and ventilation. Maureen said that the clinic was going to have it set up, but it had not happened yet. The doctor needed to order it, but she was not certain if this had already been done. I let her know that I would call the clinic in the morning, as it was past five p.m., and the clinic had already closed.

We returned to Faith in the living room. She looked exhausted and worn. She agreed to have a personal support worker and a referral to hospice for a volunteer to come into the home and provide some respite. She did not want a hospital bed, but thought maybe a bed positioning wedge might work. I reassured her that we would do all we could to keep her in her home and comfortable. She seemed satisfied that everything was being taken care of and was relieved to know she would be able to stay home rather than go to hospital.

Before I left the room, she smiled, wrote something down on her paper, and handed it to me: "It was nice to meet you." I thought that was so considerate of her. I also thought that maybe, somewhere and somehow in these two and a half hours, I had done something right. Just maybe my words or actions had reassured her and facilitated her passage from this life to the next. Faith did not want much and her sister did not want much. The idea that she could die in her own home meant the most to both. There was a huge sigh of relief. It was as if that was all they needed to know. The rest would work itself out.

At the door, I said goodbye to Maureen, who was thankful for everything. I told her I would come again. She knew how to get in touch with me and who to call after hours.

The next morning, as soon as I got into the office, I left a message for the visiting nurse, asking her to ensure that she discussed and obtained the DNR. I called the Palliative Care Network to request that they help me find a local palliative care physician. I called two different doctors directly. Neither was able to take over her care. One had too many palliatives already, and the other wasn't in the same geographical area as Faith. I put a call in to a third doctor and left a message for a callback. In the meantime, I called the ALS clinic with an update on the client's status. I made sure that the oxygen would be set up in the home then I left the office to do another home visit that afternoon.

The next day when I arrived at work, there was an urgent message from one of the case managers working with the support team. The nursing staff on the support team cover calls when we are out of the office doing home visits. She informed me that Faith had died the evening before. There was other information about the situation, and I pulled up the electronic file. I was anxious to talk to her directly. I had a lot of respect for this colleague's abilities and was happy that she was the one who had taken the call. When she worked in the community we had a "buddy system" and we covered each other's caseloads. We both understood how the other worked.

When I spoke with her, she told me that Maureen had called the office the night before. She remembered Maureen was soft spoken and very calm. Maureen informed her that Faith had died five minutes before. Maureen said she was by her side and her death was peaceful. Following policy, the Support Team case manager determined that the nurse had discussed DNR, and Faith had agreed that she did not want to be resuscitated. Maureen was there when it had been discussed. Support called the nursing agency to tell them what had transpired. The agency sent a nurse out to pronounce the death.

I spoke with Maureen a few days later. She was very calm. She was grateful that things had gone as smoothly as they did, though she missed her sister terribly!

Initially, Maureen and Faith were both struggling with a diagnosis that was new to them. Faith had been unwell for a while, but the diagnosis was relatively new. Over a short period of time they came to trust the health care providers. They were calm and did not want much in the way of care. There was a discussion about personal support workers, which they did agree to have involved. Maureen was an amazing support to her sister. They had a mutual care and respect for each other. They were happy with the support provided. The most important thing was that Faith stay at home to die and this is what happened.

A Graceful Journey
Wendy's Story

Throughout my nursing career, I have been very fortunate. I have experienced many unique situations and have many memories. In this short story, I will describe an event I feel so honoured to have been present for. It touched my heart and stayed with me all these years.

Years ago, when I was working as a visiting nurse, I visited a palliative care patient to assess her pain and symptom management and provide support. The patient, Vivian, was living with her daughter. When I did the visit, she was in bed and was extremely short of breath. Vivian told me that her granddaughter's birthday was coming up in a couple of days and she wanted to be present for the event. Her granddaughter was turning seven years old. On the day of my visit, her granddaughter was at school. Vivian's wishes were to remain in her daughter's home for as long as she could before transferring to hospital for her final journey.

As I was completing Vivian's nursing assessment, I realized she was in severe respiratory distress and had rales [abnormal respiratory sounds] throughout both her lungs. As I was speaking with Vivian to assess her condition, she said she was comfortable, but her breathing was an issue. She reiterated that she really wanted to be present for her granddaughter's birthday in two more days. I asked Vivian's daughter, Susan, to check if Vivian had any Lasix or other diuretic, which she had been taking on occasion. Susan looked in the medicine basket where she kept all Vivian's medications. There was no diuretic or Lasix. My thought was if the patient was able to take a diuretic medication for her respiratory failure, it might resolve enough so she would be able to stay in her home comfortably until her granddaughter's birthday.

I picked up the phone and contacted Vivian's family doctor. I gave him an update on Vivian's present health status and her wish to stay at home for a couple more days. I advocated for Vivian to stay home longer, as she requested, and the physician agreed. He ordered some Lasix for Vivian and said he was faxing the script to the local pharmacy as we spoke. His plan was to do a home visit later in the day to see Vivian. After I hung up the phone, I went into Vivian's room and spoke with her and Susan to share the plan with them. They were pleased. I asked if someone could go to the pharmacy and pick up the medication for Vivian. I told them I would stay until she had taken her medication and she was more settled.

Both Vivian and her daughter thanked me. Susan said her nephew was coming to visit within the hour. She would call him and ask him to pick up the medication at the local pharmacy. In the meantime, Vivian wanted to have a little rest as she was feeling exhausted. I made sure she was comfortable in her bed and went out to the kitchen to document the events of the visit in her chart.

After sitting in the kitchen and charting for a few minutes, there was a knock on the front door. Susan went to answer it. It was her brother, Bob, and his wife, Sheila. Susan was shocked to see them. They were not expected to arrive for a couple of days, as they were planning to attend her daughter's birthday party. After greeting Bob and Sheila, she introduced them to me. Then they went in to see Vivian.

Vivian woke up. When she saw Bob, she had tears in her eyes. He went over to her and gave her a big hug. She was thrilled and all smiles to see him. Susan explained to me that Bob was her mom's favourite child. The family made a semi-circle around Vivian's bed, holding hands with each other and Vivian. This allowed Vivian to speak softly to them. She was very short of breath but was able to tell each one how much she loved them and how happy and proud she was of each of them. After her words to them, they each came closer to her and hugged her and told her how much they loved her. Bob was the last to hug her and tell her how much he loved her and how much she meant to him. Vivian gave a final breath and passed away in his arms.

I was standing at the doorway and was in awe of the beautiful scene. Bob looked at me and started to cry. "I think she is gone," he whispered. I slipped over quietly to the side of Vivian's bed and checked for breathing and her pulse. I looked at her family and said, "Yes, she is at peace now." As the family gathered and hugged each other in their loss of Vivian, her grandson arrived at the house with the medication. He was just moments too late.

As a nurse, this was an experience I will never forget. It was a gift for me to witness Vivian's graceful journey while she passed away with her family by her side. I knew her wishes were fulfilled, and I knew I had been privileged to have a small part in that journey.

Wendy is an experienced and skilled nurse. As a seasoned nurse, she has medical knowledge, knowledge of herself, and at the visit she gains knowledge of her patient and the patient's family. Wendy was able to support the patient and family through her own comfort with the illness, treatments, and the dying process. She identified the patient's wishes and stayed with the patient and family until the end, helping them through the transition. This was a powerful encounter. The needs of the patient, family, and nurse were met.

FRONT LINE NURSING STORIES

New to Palliative Care
Laurie's Story

As I mentioned at the start of this chapter, the foundation of nursing is science. To graduate, nurses need to have basic knowledge essential for practice. This is then complemented by ongoing learning that takes place in practice or in courses and workshops that nurses attend to build on their skills. They identify gaps in knowledge and come up with ways to fill those gaps and improve the knowledge and skills they already have. At graduation, nurses generally are at the "novice" level. Science coupled with experience brings an ease to the practice setting, whereby art can emerge. As nurses gain experience and learn new skills, in time they can become "expert" nurses in their chosen area of practice.

I sat down with two visiting nurses to talk about their experiences in the community. It was interesting to watch and listen, and the interaction is worth sharing. I already knew Deb, who was a seasoned nurse, and I was meeting Laurie, a novice nurse, for the first time. They talked about palliative care. Deb sat and listened to Laurie tell her stories. Then she shared some insights and a story of her own.

As a visiting nurse, I have only had limited experience with palliative care. I have to say that I have been blessed. The first patients and families I cared for were very calm and supportive of each other.

The first palliative lady I cared for had her daughter with her twenty-four hours a day. The daughter was very receptive to any kind of recommendations. Pain control was the main issue. If it was under control, things were fine. The patient's decline happened quickly. There were not a lot of symptoms, but the patient did require the symptom relief kit (SRK).

Taking care of this patient and family was a valuable experience for me. I was able to tap into my nurse colleagues for support. They were more experienced and very informative. I could ask them for input on how to approach things. I wanted the best for my patient and her family and wanted to be sure

205

they got the support they needed during the dying process. I needed to put a port into place so that medications could be administered that route. They supported me with that. I remember that when I needed to teach the family about the SRK, my colleagues coached me on the conversation leading up to the use of the kit. They reminded me that learning to do this was often intimidating for families. Usually this was because families were fearful that they might cause harm to the person they loved. It was a matter of me finding a way to encourage families and give them the support and confidence to do what they needed to do to care for their loved one.

My first palliative lady had chronic obstructive lung disease (COPD). She died peacefully at home. When this happened, I had one of my more experienced nurse colleagues do the home visit to pronounce the death. This lady was an ideal patient for me to take care of, as it was my initial experience dealing with death. I did a lot of reflective practice with that patient and family. My fear was that the patient and family would be looking to me for support and that I might not be able to give them what they needed. They communicated well with me. They let me know what their needs were and what fears or concerns they had. This way, I was able to answer questions and support them appropriately. It was a calm environment. They were grieving and knew they were grieving. They supported each other in their grief.

In my most recent experience, it was important for me to understand how much the family wanted to be involved. The daughter was the caregiver. She also worked as a personal support worker in the community. She was quite devoted to her mother and did a lot for her. I needed to remember how much she needed to be involved each step of the way. She wanted me to know and act accordingly.

Before palliative care, her mother had been on service for a long time because of a stroke. She required catheter changes by the nurse, as well as other things. Eventually, her mother's condition deteriorated, and slowly she became palliative. Her daughter was very worried about giving her the pain medication. I reviewed what was in the SRK and reassured her that she could have a port in place so that her mother would not feel the needle prick each time she was given something for pain. In her own way, she told me what she needed. I listened to her cues. The daughter initially did not think she needed frequent visits. When pain was an issue, she was grateful to have the teaching and guidance about the medications. She learned when and how to use them. It worked for them.

Laurie told me how she often communicated with her mentor, Deb. She told me what she said and did to get affirmation or suggestions on how to do better when working with palliative patients. Laurie emphasized the importance of reflection, especially with palliative patients. She would ask herself: Did I do all I could do? Did I say what needed to be said? Am I giving them all that they need? What can I learn from this without beating myself up too much for what I could have done better? Deb remarked that she still asks those same sorts of questions all the time. "These are good questions to ask... and reflecting is a good thing to do. It should never go away."

Palliative Care: Sometimes it Is More Complex
Deb's Story

Deb laughed and remarked that she is a person with a lot of different personalities. She said, "I am one person, but there are many parts to me. I pull out the various parts as the situation presents itself... I am not always the same person with everyone. It depends on what is needed." She told us that this approach generally worked, as she didn't fall into too many "pits."

Not only do I change, but the frequency of my visits change, depending on what the need is at the time. If we are moving along as things need to be, then I back off and reduce my visits. Other times, I might have to visit twice a day. It all depends on what needs to be accomplished and where we are with things. If things are going well, then I back off. When the nurse goes to visit people who are sick, the patient is reminded of their disease and all that is wrong. The focus then is on the illness and not the other things in life.

Sometimes, people need to just live and not be reminded of what is going badly or what is happening with the illness. I build my frequency and tempo depending on what they need and where we need to go at the time. Some days, I call the person up, and if they are doing fine, then I will cancel the visit for that day. Other times, I may spend extra time talking with them about their family or something important to them. This builds rapport and reenergizes.

The person that comes to mind and who I want to tell you about is a palliative care patient I had a few months ago. I am a visiting nurse in the community and do direct care. I was the second nurse to visit. It had been requested that I do the visit as a symptom relief kit was sent into the home. I needed to review this with the family. I was told the diagnosis was breast cancer. I called and spoke with the husband the night before and booked my visit for the next afternoon. I thought the time would be better, as I wouldn't be as rushed and could spend some extra time with the family.

I went into the home, but didn't know what to expect. I had a nursing student with me. This had been cleared with the spouse the night before. When I walked into the home, the tension was so thick. I thought I could cut it with a knife. I introduced myself and my student and sat down at the kitchen table. The patient's daughter introduced herself to me. She would have been in her late thirties or early forties. She was sitting in the chair, red in the face, and very tense. I could see she was trying to relax but couldn't manage it. She proceeded to tell me how she had been texting the physician.

Then the patient's husband came into the room. I was facing the daughter, and the husband came into the room and stood behind me. He was talking and sounded quite angry. He was talking to me. His sentences were short and abrupt. It dawned on me that the patient's spouse and daughter had been arguing. I assumed that my arrival interrupted what had been going on. The reason for my visit was to teach the family about the SRK and how and when to use the medications in the kit. They were not interested in talking about the patient's pain or the medication use.

I pulled out the patient's chart that was in the home and started looking at it. It showed that there was cancer of the breast with brain metastasis. I was trying to get a sense of things and asked if the patient was able to join us in the kitchen. They said she couldn't and that she needed help to get out of bed and get to the commode. She had just been admitted to service, but it was my view that she was admitted to service late in the diagnosis. She was cascading to end-of-life status.

The atmosphere at the table was getting tense. The husband didn't want to look me in the face. He and the daughter were starring angrily at each other. I was trying to understand what was going on in there.

I decided I needed to meet the patient. I told them I needed to go into her room to meet her. I invited one of them to join me. Her daughter came with me. The husband stayed out. On the way to the room, I learned that the spouse held the power of attorney (POA) for personal care. The daughter whispered this to me on the way to the room. She also told me that he was her stepfather, as her mother had remarried.

I wear hearing aids and I couldn't understand half of what she was whispering, but I could tell by her body language she wasn't happy. I trailed behind her as she guided me down the hall. The fact that the spouse was POA was important to know. He would be the one to make decisions for the patient when she could no longer do this herself.

When we got to her room, the patient opened her eyes, said a word or two. It was obvious she couldn't grasp everything that was going on around her. I asked about the pain and "yes," she was having pain lying there, and it was worse with movements. Her daughter reported that she cried out and grimaced when they tried to lift her up or turn her. I asked where and was told the pain was worse in her legs. I wondered if she had cancer in the bones and was told she had bone metastasis. I got more information about her pain and what I could do to manage it. I had not reviewed her medications yet. I did her vitals. Her blood pressure was elevated. I could see she had thrush in her mouth, so swallowing was a bit of a problem. I wasn't sure if it was because she was actively dying or because of her use of Decadron (medication to relieve inflammation). I would need to deal with that. She was on hydromorphone for pain, at a low dose but not enough, as it was even too painful for her to get off the toilet.

We returned to the kitchen table and her daughter showed me a pain diary. For the last two days, they had been keeping track of the amount of the medication her mother was using. Her daughter said she had already texted the information to the physician. There was a plan to talk with the doctor the next day. They would review the information and look at increasing the dose of the long-acting medication. I was a bit surprised that they were texting each other.

I needed to do a full admission assessment, but also needed to address her lack of adequate pain control before we could talk about other things. Lack of pain control was causing other things to escalate. We reviewed the dosage of medications and added up the extra pain medication used, as her pain was out of control. I asked her daughter to continue giving the pain medication, as it was helping. I also asked her to consider giving her mom medication for breakthrough pain a half hour before she needed to do any treatment. I explained that her legs were giving her mother pain; if she had to get up to go to the bathroom or turn in the bed, then it hurt. I explained that standing on her legs or moving was causing bone pain, and this needed to be addressed. I let the daughter know that she could really make a difference today if she could start to anticipate the things that were giving her mom pain. She could treat her ahead of time and it would not be so hard for her to manage. This was a little something that I could offer them. I told them that we would look at the SRK the next day. I let her know that meanwhile, if she needed, she could call the agency in the night. She could let them know she had already had the SRK. She could, if necessary, ask for them to make a home visit for support. I told her that the nurse would understand what that means. They had the tools and they had the number to call if they needed.

I left the visit and said I would be back the next day. After I walked out of the home, I turned to my student and said, "My goodness, was I imagining things or was it terrible in there?"

She said, "Oh yeah, there is something going on."

A lot happened, but I will try to keep my story brief. The family intended to keep the patient home throughout her illness. Their preference was for her to die at home. Residential hospice was not seen to be an option. They wanted to look after her at home.

The daughter had taken a leave of absence from work. She wasn't living there but was there most of the time. She did not like her stepfather. She didn't want anything to do with him. They were competing over what to do for her mother's plan of care and decision-making.

The patient's daughter was reaching out to the physician for support. The spouse was upset with the physician. The spouse felt that the physician had not made the diagnosis fast enough when the cancer first started a couple of years earlier. He felt the diagnosis was missed and the cancer had advanced to Stage Four. He believed it could have been stopped earlier. He wanted nothing to do with the physician. He had the POA and did not want to talk with the physician.

So here was the daughter, texting back and forth with the physician. And here I was, caught in between. I was trying to take care of and provide the best for my patient. I was trying to get the daughter and patient's spouse to cooperate with each other in order to take care of my patient.

When we left the house, I told the student, "I have three patients in there, not one." She laughed and understood. She had witnessed it and experienced it herself. They both loved this woman. They just couldn't stand each other.

I did the visit the next morning. At this time, we had all the numbers. We worked things out. We increased the patient's pain medication and dealt with her pain. It started to improve. I got orders to treat her mouth and did the things nurses do: looked after the business, anticipated she would need a catheter, and got an order for it to be used as needed.

When I showed the daughter and the spouse the symptom relief kit, I showed them the Haldol it contained, which is used to reduce anxiety. Because of her brain metastasis, I anticipated that we could give the patient as much Decadron as she needed, but she was probably going to have confusion and anxiety. The spouse was certainly going to have anxiety. We wanted to control her anxiety and, hence, her spouse's anxiety. This was important to help the patient and family manage at home. I showed them the Haldol and told them what it would be used for. I told them we would be there every day or possibly twice a day. The pain issue was addressed, and we addressed the thrush. She was still eating, but I needed to talk with her spouse and daughter about nutrition and let them know what to expect and how that was going to change. It was a busy visit.

The husband did not want to increase her pain medication. He felt that it would make her foggy. If that happened, then he felt he would not be able to connect with her. The patient's husband wasn't getting past his own issues. He wasn't looking at what her needs were. He was looking at what he needed and wanted. He was trying to keep her home with him physically and mentally just as long as he could. The daughter was picking up on what was happening.

She wanted the pain controlled. The daughter had her own agenda. She was experiencing grief that she wasn't dealing with. The patient's daughter did a lot of the personal care. She guided the personal support workers when they were there. The spouse didn't want his wife to move around too much because of the pain.

I had to do a lot of teaching in that home with the patient's family. I worked hard to get the spouse on board. I tried to explain things logically so he could understand what I was doing. He had to get to know me and he had to get to trust me. He had to see that his goals were my goals. In order to manage each symptom, I had to get his cooperation to bring him forward. It came to a point where we needed to start subcutaneous medication, as the patient couldn't take oral medications. She needed to go on a pump. I started to do the intermittent hydromorphone, because it was fast. I said we should put a button in, and when we were ready to do her care, we could give her a hit. When he saw good results, he agreed. We had to keep up her Decadron. I got the physician to order that subcutaneously. We showed her husband how to do that. This way, he was able to do something directly to help her. We had to start the Haldol subcutaneously at some point.

Related to all this, it was interesting that the patient's physician called me one morning at about eight-thirty a.m., as I was sitting in my car doing some paperwork. He asked me if I was going in to see her. I told him I was planning on it. He said he had been in contact with the daughter. He needed to get a pump in place, as the patient was trying to chew her pills. He told me he spoke to the husband, who didn't want any part of it. The physician told me that the husband did not want any part of interacting with him, either. He said, "We need to get this pump going, and I am wondering if you can do that." I agreed. He asked me to call him on his cell when it was done.

The husband was an angry man. I knew he did not want any part of interacting with the physician. I already knew that he didn't want anything to do with the pump. Through reasoning with him, I was able to get his consent.

Eventually, the patient didn't want to get out of bed. She was incontinent and we needed to put the catheter in. Her husband didn't want that. I turned her over in bed and showed him her wet bottom and the reddened areas on her skin. I explained that if her skin got worse, she would have more pain, a different pain, a pain that she didn't really need to have. I said to him, "Let us put a really small catheter in place and we can see how it goes. If it bothers her, we can take it out." He wasn't on board until I could give him options and he could decide. He was very controlling.

This was a very complex situation. If I could get my patient cared for properly, I didn't care. I needed to figure out the patient's family. When I could do that, then I could look after her and my goals were met. My goals were to provide care and support for my patient.

After my visits, the daughter would often follow me out to the car. She had her own needs. She needed information and support, and she needed to vent. One day, she followed me outside in the winter and she was in tears. I listened and then was very direct and told her she needed to reach out and talk with someone about her grief. She felt helpless and needed support. I started working with the family and their grief at an early stage.

My patient died on a weekend when I was off. Her daughter let me know. The physician only made a couple of visits during the whole dying process. It was just too difficult for him to be in that home. It was too tense, and the husband was difficult and angry. This patient situation was more complicated than some. I kept the case manager updated on things and had her support. It ended up being a very peaceful death, and my patient's pain was controlled. The daughter and spouse were both grieving in different ways. In the end, I did have a feeling of accomplishment.

Once the death occurs, I don't keep in contact with the family. That is the end of the relationship. I am not an expert in the grieving process, so I suggest and let them know that there is help for them through that stage.

I have been doing this type of work in the community for years. I work from a science base, and it is a downfall of our system that when we go into the home to provide direct care, we have very limited information. I was blindsided. When I went to see the patient initially, I didn't know she had brain or bone metastasis. It is a problem with the system. I needed to be a nurse, psychologist, social worker, all rolled into one to meet the challenge.

Deb is an expert nurse working with palliative patients. She has a lot of practical experience, and it means a lot. She has the knowledge, skills, and confidence to work with the patient, family, physician, and case manager. She can identify the barriers to her providing the patient with the care needed.

She finds strategies to deal with each of them. In this way, she can ensure the patient is kept comfortable.

Deb notes: "Palliative care is sometimes more complex." When she left the home after her first visit, she pointed out to the student that she "had three patients and not one." She knows the importance of understanding the patient within the context of family. Deb also reminds us that nurses are always learning, including herself.

Things to Consider
Marian's Story

Ruth was in her late forties. She lived on the lake in a two-story cottage with her husband and their two schnauzers. The couple did not have any children and had very few supports in the area.

I made the home visit to assess her needs. She had recently been admitted to the community program with a diagnosis of breast cancer that had metastasized to her bones and lungs. Ruth's cancer was end-stage. There was a percutaneous catheter in place to drain fluid that accumulated in the pleural cavity of her lung. She had a dressing on her chest area. The visiting nurses were doing drain/wound care and palliative care, which included pain and symptom management.

When I made the visit, the dogs barked like mad when I rang the bell. Schnauzers are known to be protective animals, and these two were very excited. I am partial to schnauzers. They are so cute, with their whiskered snouts and bushy eyebrows. These two were both salt-and-pepper colour. We had owned a schnauzer for years, so I was also familiar with their temperament.

Gordon, the spouse, called the dogs away with authority. He seemed a bit worried about the situation and noise they were creating. He had a firm voice with them. They listened to him when he instructed them to stop and calm down. He put them in a room on the main floor of the house. I let him know about our own dog and my soft spot for schnauzers. He seemed to relax and brought me upstairs to the bedroom, where Ruth was sitting quietly in an armchair.

Ruth had a medium build, with auburn hair and fair skin. She was frail, soft-spoken but confident. We talked briefly about the dogs. It was obvious that they loved their pets. My affection for the dogs was genuine, and I believe they sensed it.

The couple both seemed tense. Gordon let Ruth do most of the talking. As I completed the home visit, it was apparent that Ruth had not done much planning about her future. There was an opening in our conversation where I asked about her palliative state. She told me she knew she was palliative. I asked about a do-not-resuscitate (DNR) order and whether she had one in place. She did not have one. I explained what it was exactly and that it did not mean she would not have treatment. The DNR meant that if her heart stopped, the staff would not perform chest compressions to get her heart going again. We talked more about it. She confidently told me that she wanted to have a DNR in place. She didn't want any heroics, should her heart stop. I completed the paperwork.

Talking about this led to a discussion about where she would like to be in her last stages of dying, and when the time was right. She had Gordon and a couple of close friends and a few distant relatives. She did not have a very large support network. I talked about the options and what services we could provide in the home. Her preference was to go to hospice, although she had not yet been to see one. I talked about the local hospice and what she could expect. I encouraged the couple to book a visit there. They said they would do that. Gordon thought it was great that he would be able to bring the dogs over for visits. He knew he would have to be responsible for them.

As we talked about the issues, both Ruth and Gordon started to relax. Some of the tension I sensed when I arrived was dissipating. At the end of my visit, Ruth thanked me for coming and for talking with her about all the things we had discussed. She told me that no one had talked with her about these issues, and she was relieved and happy that this had happened today. It was as if a large weight had been lifted from her shoulders.

It is important to meet the person where they are. In this situation, there was an opening and an opportunity to learn more about what Ruth knew about her condition and to discuss planning for her death. Ruth's condition was deteriorating, and although it can be a difficult conversation, it is an important one. There can be a risk if the person is not yet ready to talk about it. When this happens, the person usually finds a way to shut that conversation down. In this case, Ruth was very appreciative and extremely relieved.

10. Challenges to Overcome

Rough-and-Tumble Men
Kerry's Story

I have worked as a nurse doing both oncology and palliative care. This is a story that, unless I do something very different between now and when I retire, will be the most profound experience I have ever had in nursing.

I tend to have a soft spot in my heart for what I call "rough-and-tumble men of the woods." They are the older males who often live isolated, alone, in a wilderness-type setting. These are men who have a cabin in the woods without much support, and they are lucky if they have running water. These ones creep into my heart. I truly don't know why this is, because I try to give the best to all my patients. Somehow, I seem to take these ones under my wings and try to do for them. What I appreciate about them is that their life doesn't stop because they have a life-limiting diagnosis. These are the men who go on no matter what.

I remember one fellow in his eighties who collected scrap metal. This was a man with rectal cancer, out every day in his car, picking up scrap metal. He was out there, trying to make a buck to get his next meal. He had so much rectal pain and yet he continued. When I got him a ROHO cushion, he thought he was in seventh heaven, driving around on this special cushion. It made him so happy to have this pressure relief on his rectum. It meant he could continue to maintain his financial status longer. These fellows are very resourceful and hardy. They can manage with very limited supports. I think it is that aspect that draws me to them.

The gentleman that I really want to tell you about is Steve. He was another one of my rough-and-tumble men of the woods. He was about seventy years old, of German descent, and he didn't speak English all that well. The first challenge was recognizing that his English was limited. The initial assessment ended up taking me three home visits to complete. I didn't find out till I got there how difficult communication would be. We worked through it. We made signs and basically played charades to exchange information. Then I decided to get a professional interpreter who could speak German to come out with me to do the visits.

Steve had come to Canada on his own twenty-five years earlier. He had left his family in Germany. He had two children and was separated from his wife. I didn't know this initially, but found out later that he was estranged from his family.

When I met Steve, he had been diagnosed with non-Hodgkin's lymphoma. He was getting chemotherapy and had come on service for nursing to help manage the side effects of his treatment and disease process. He was having a huge issue with pain control and was trying to get a narcotic that wouldn't constipate him so much that he would end up with nausea, vomiting, and constipation so bad that he couldn't, in his own words, "take a dump."

The other problem with Steve was that finances were so tight he couldn't afford the medication he needed. The doctor gave him some Cymbalta on a trial basis, and it worked. The doctor wanted to put him on Cymbalta for his neuropathic pain. There were the two components of his pain: he needed both a neuropathic pain relief agent and a regular narcotic. The Cymbalta was $135 for a prescription that only lasted thirty days. The combination of Cymbalta and Tramacet worked, and Steve was so happy to get some pain relief and "take a dump." This was before he knew how much it cost.

I ended up calling the family doctor to see if he could get some free samples of Cymbalta from the pharmaceutical representative that Steve could use. Sure enough, this is what he did. Steve and I used to laugh when I said to him that I was his "drug runner." He would let me know when he was low, and I would stop off at the doctor's office, get him more free samples, and bring them to his house. He didn't drive, so he had difficulty with transportation. He had difficulty with practically every part of his life. He had no money, no transportation, and no supports. He had nobody.

The next thing was that he couldn't see to read the information I would bring him, like pamphlets about side effects of medications and what he could do. The translator would help me get things translated into German, but he couldn't read it. He couldn't afford an eye exam. We then solicited help. I called different optical places in our area, and one of them said they would give him the "gift of life" if I could get him in there to see them. This meant having to get him to his appointment. Arrangements were made through the local hospice for a volunteer to bring him to his appointment, and he was given free glasses. This way he could at least read the information he was given and be informed of things.

He had an occupational therapist for equipment, and a social worker became involved to help with planning related to a will and power of attorney. I was starting to feel like a social worker myself, and it was taking up a lot of my time to work on many of the things that needed to be addressed. I knew the social worker would be valuable for him in order to get through some of these challenges. He had difficulties with the town about his water and a culvert that was out by the road in front of his property. The water would back up in the culvert and then into his property and his house. He had difficulty communicating and representing himself. He needed help to get through some of these issues and work with the city to resolve them. It was worked out that the social worker would advocate for him on a few fronts.

The nurse involved who did the direct care was fabulous. She worked in the northern community and was known to often go above and beyond. Steve's treatment for lymphoma wasn't working any longer. With lymphoma, bleeding, infection, and anemia are all issues. At the end, one of these takes over. We then needed to look at an end-of-life plan for Steve. That is when Steve divulged that he had left Germany twenty-five years earlier and that he was estranged from his wife and children.

What he wanted was to go back to Germany and for me to help him get back there so he could reunite with his family and die there. That was not going to happen. He was unable to fly at this point. The bleeding and infection risks were too much. He had already been having infections. Through talking with him, I discovered that the most important thing was for him to connect with his family. It was not necessarily being back there, where he had no place to stay. For him, it was more important for him to connect than to be physically there with his family.

This is when I got Gerda involved. She is a support person who works with the same agency as I do but in a different role. She is an assistant in our organization who is German and speaks German. The next thing was to track down his family. The organization that we worked for was not supportive in this endeavour, so this was something I needed to do on my own time.

The goal was to locate his family and set up a Skype call so Steve could connect. Steve had no Internet connection, so that would be a challenge. I approached the agency management, as I knew we had web cams and knew we weren't using them at the time. I asked if I could borrow a computer to set up Skype to connect this gentleman who was "end of life" with his family overseas. I explained the significance it had for him as he was dying. I was told that they did not have a policy and procedure in place yet to lend out web cams or computers. The bottom line is that it wasn't something they could do.

I went back to the palliative care team as I did every week for rounds. Part of my role was to work with this team for our palliative and end-of-life patients who wanted this intervention. I mentioned Steve's wishes to Connie, the hospice case manager, and told her the challenges we were having. She said she had a computer with Skype on it and offered to lend it to us. This was in the early days of Skype, when it was quite new. She said she would work with us on her own time to make this happen for Steve.

While I was doing footwork here, Gerda was doing online searches to find Steve's family. She had their names and last known whereabouts as a starting point. They weren't living there anymore, but she did come up with a name which matched that of Steve's son. Gerda was able to find the son. When she connected with him, he confirmed that his father had left Europe many years earlier. He was so overwhelmed that someone was calling him from the other side of the world to say his father was searching for him. Then he learned that his father's health was poor and that he wanted to connect with the family before he passed away. The son told Gerda that his sister was alive and well and lived close by. He told her that Steve had grandchildren. Gerda recorded the names and birthdates of all the grandchildren for Steve.

The next task was to get an internet provider involved to help make Skype possible. I needed to go over to Rogers to see if they could help me. I explained that Steve had no internet. The company sent a fellow out to Steve's place who was just fabulous. He was a young guy in his late twenties. I told him I would meet him at the patient's home. He knew there was no cable or internet access and that his job was to connect Steve. He said to me, "Don't you worry. I'm in on this and it isn't going to cost you a cent." This young guy then climbed a very tall pole and attached something. He said the people in the area would be shocked to find they could get free movies while we got Steve connected to Skype. It took him two hours to get things connected. We were so excited and so grateful.

It was important to do a trial run to be sure it would work. I have very little technology expertise, and Connie had only a bit more than me. We were doing this all on our own time after work. We did a trial run on Family Day, February 15, 2009. We chose that day because this is a statutory holiday for us, and we could all be there at the same time. Several weeks had gone by before we could get all this orchestrated. In the meantime, Steve had been conversing with his son on the phone at different intervals.

The Skype call ended up happening on a Saturday or Sunday morning. Steve was at home in his hospital bed. Gerda and Connie were there with me, as was the Rogers guy. A neighbour from down the road came over with an electric razor to get Steve shaved up, nice and presentable. We got him connected and we left him with his family while we went into the next room. We wanted to give him privacy, but we could hear him. Where I was sitting, I could see him. Tears were streaming down his face while he visited with them by Skype. The family was crying, and he was crying, and so were we. It was the most profound thing I have ever experienced. It was the joy of this family reconnecting after so long. Who knows what had happened so long ago? The pure joy!

Steve's son and daughter and their spouses were there. The grandchildren were all there and got introduced one by one. They spent a good hour talking and chatting. I couldn't understand the words, but I could see and feel the emotion. Once they were finished and said their goodbyes, we gave Steve a few minutes on his own. We could hear him sobbing in the room. When we went into his room, he was laughing. He said thank you to us and told us how important that was to him.

The next day, I got a call from the nurse to say that he wasn't doing well. He was bleeding, so an ambulance was called to take him to hospital. He passed away the next day.

This gave us the opportunity to call his family and let them know he passed away. We packed up his watch and ring and the very few possessions he owned. We sent them to his family so they had something of their dad after he died.

As far as friends, he'd told me that he had a lot of friends who would call him when they wanted help with things at their house that needed to be done. He told me he had friends who liked to drink his homemade wine. Friends that "like to drink and carry on and want me to help them do things in their house."

Steve had a wild cat that he had taken in. When he was alive, he fed the cat and attended to it. For a few days after he died, Terri, the nurse, one of the neighbours, and I took turns going over to feed the cat and let it in and out of the house.

Some neighbours noticed that a couple of Steve's fair-weather friends had been seen trying to get into Steve's home. It was thought that they were trying to get in so they could go through his stuff and help themselves to anything of value. I called the police and told them what had happened. They were very supportive. They drove to his home regularly and circled his place to make sure that these so-called friends stayed away.

The family took the time to send us an email after Steve died. It was written in German and Gerda translated it for us. I haven't told this story once where I have been able to get through it without crying. There were so many people who came together on their own time to make this happen for Steve. It is the true meaning of team and getting a whole team to wrap itself around the patient and make sure his end of life went well. No one person could have done this without the other people doing their piece. This is the reward we get and that is what keeps me going. It is the response from family and patients. It is knowing that you have made a difference in their life.

11. Ethics in Brief

Ethics refers to the concept of right or wrong conduct. All people have their own ethical principles (i.e., honesty, respect, personal responsibility) that they use to guide them in their daily living. They allow us to judge our own behaviour. Ethics deals with issues of morality, rules of behaviour, and moral correctness of conduct.

Registered nurses have a code of ethics for the profession. Each nurse is obliged to observe this ethical standard. There are nursing values and ethical principles within the code of ethics. The code provides a means for self-evaluation, feedback, and peer review. It also serves as a base from which nurses advocate for quality practice environments that support the delivery of safe, compassionate, competent, and ethical care.[2]

The following stories illustrate how the issues that come up in nursing can be challenging or complex. As nurses we are forced to examine our own values, the values of the patient, family and team, the code of ethics of the profession, and general ethical principles. Some situations call for a more in-depth examination and gathering of the facts, and sometimes there is a need to determine which ethical principles are in conflict and explore possible options and an action plan.

The following nursing stories merely touch on the concept of ethics.

---

2   The Code of Ethics for Registered Nurses is available on the Canadian Nurses Association website: https://cna-aiic.ca/en/nursing-practice/nursing-ethics

MARIAN FACCIOLO

Who Am I to Judge You?
Stephanie's Story

At the age of forty-eight, Patrick was young to have suffered a stroke. The agency I worked for had just set up a program where people with new strokes would receive treatment and rehab at the hospital and then have a preplanned discharge from hospital to home. Prior to this, people leaving the acute care setting of the hospital after a stroke might end up waiting a year or two, and sometimes longer, to get in-home therapy services. Early intervention with stroke victims is very important.

With the new program, there would be a case conference at the hospital prior to discharge. The hospital team would meet with the community partners to come up with a plan of care prior to discharge. I was notified of the time and meeting place at the local hospital. Patrick and his wife, Lisa, would be in attendance.

When I arrived for the conference, the community occupational therapist, hospital discharge planner, hospital case manager, and hospital therapists were all there. Patrick came into the room. He was a stocky man with a shaved head and beard. I was introduced to him and his wife, Lisa. When Patrick spoke, he sounded gruff and rough around the edges.

Patrick had worked as a plumber before this stroke. To resume this type of work would require him to have a higher level of cognitive function and retraining. Physically, he had lost strength and balance, but it was thought that with intensive retraining, he would be able to improve significantly. After his stroke, he did use a walker for a short while. He would go home with a cane because his mobility had improved while he was in hospital. A bath aid was rented for use at home so that he could be safe when bathing.

On Patrick's discharge from hospital, arrangements were made for an occupational therapist for his cognitive retraining; a physiotherapist for strength training and safety with mobility; a social worker to facilitate community integration, help with coping, link with financial resources and assist with lifestyle changes; a nurse to teach about the illness and medication management, smoking cessation and lifestyle changes; and a speech language pathologist to work closely with him on issues related to his speech and cognition.

It wasn't long after our initial meeting that Patrick went home. I met with him and his wife within days of his return and completed a detailed home assessment. It was difficult going into the home, because I felt that I was walking into a smokestack. Both smoked heavily. They told me they each smoked between one and a half to two packs a day. Patrick had quit since his stroke. He was finding it difficult to be around Lisa's smoking. Lisa smoked outside, close to the house. It was hard to tell that this was the case, as the house reeked of stale smoke.

The couple owned a dog. He was a large, overly friendly collie that shed all over the house. The couches were covered with thick dog hair. The dog loved visitors and jumped up at me whenever I visited. He would sniff and nuzzle his snout into my private area. This behaviour didn't seem to bother Patrick or Lisa. They said he was their "baby" and excused him by saying, "He just likes people. He's just being affectionate." It always puzzled me why they didn't ask him to stop jumping or sniffing. That really bothered me.

As a team, we had many conferences with Patrick at his home. At some point, it became evident that Patrick was not going to change his lifestyle, even though this had drastic consequences for his future. He returned to smoking and drinking. He drank during the day and sometimes before the therapist would visit. This affected his ability to do the required work with the therapist. He admitted that he loved to party, and he had a history of drug abuse and incarceration.

We really wanted to see Patrick succeed. At the initial conference, he told the providers that his goal was to work as a plumber again. To achieve this goal would require a lot of self-directed therapy between the visits from the professionals. Initially, he worked hard to do the exercises. Slowly, he resumed his past lifestyle habits. He stopped working on the program that had been designed with him to reach his goals. He struggled with making a choice. Finally, he decided to forgo the plans for therapy that he was very much involved in creating. He admitted he wasn't doing the work on his own between visits. He was sad when he shared his decision with me over the phone.

At one visit, the therapist saw a reminder about a court date on Patrick's calendar. She called me to ask if I knew anything about his being incarcerated. I did not know anything about this. This is not the type of information we would get when people were referred to our community program.

Toward the end of his time with us, Patrick returned to the local hospital by ambulance. He had lost his balance, fell and lost consciousness at home. Lisa sent him to hospital as she suspected that it might have been another stroke. Patrick lay on the stretcher in the emergency department for some time. He was triaged by the nurses and had some tests done. Once he regained consciousness, he decided he wanted to return home. The physician and nursing staff in the ER did not think he was in any state to return home. Informed of this, Patrick became belligerent, threatening to harm the hospital staff. He left the hospital against medical advice.

Once home, he called one of the therapists to tell her what had happened and to request a home visit. As the case manager, it was my responsibility to ensure the safety of all the providers. Before allowing them to go back into the home, we needed to determine that it was safe to do so. I called Patrick's family doctor to tell him about what had happened and discuss possible strategies so we could continue to work with Patrick. Each provider was informed of what had happened and was asked if they felt safe going back into the home, knowing Patrick and what had recently transpired. I notified the management team of the agency where I worked. A high-risk plan was put into place. As it turned out, none of us thought Patrick would harm us in any way. Each of us had established a therapeutic relationship with him, and we thought that he would not harm us. My own view was that if anyone was at risk, it would be me. Patrick had an issue with authority figures. It was likely that he saw me in this light, given my role.

When I think of Patrick, I think of my own biases. I haven't had a lot of exposure to people who have been convicted of criminal offenses and incarcerated. Despite this, I believe that I, like the therapists, was able to develop a therapeutic relationship with him. We all cared about who he was and how he felt. We cared about his future and actively engaged in plans that were made together with him. We all wanted Patrick to reach his goals.

After working with him for some time, we agreed that his brain injury from the stroke was such that he could not recover enough to work safely and independently as a plumber. However, we believed he could still lead a happy and dignified life if he chose to do so. I spoke to Patrick about the therapies, and it was his decision to stop having them. He told me that he felt fortunate to have had the professionals who worked so hard with him. He acknowledged that he wasn't doing his part. He knew that somewhere along the way he decided that he was not going to make the lifestyle changes required to make a difference in the potential outcomes.

During the journey with Patrick and the team, I had to identify my own biases and move forward to establish a healthy relationship that was nonjudgmental. During the risk event, I needed to analyze the situation, bring in the different people, and come up with a couple of possible plans to move forward. I trusted my instincts and those of my teammates when they wanted to proceed with the goals and plans and continue to work with him in his home environment. I don't believe we ever gave up. It was Patrick who ultimately decided his fate.

As nurses, we value the notion of providing safe, competent, and ethical care. In this case, it was also important that the people working with this patient felt safe to continue his care in the home setting. The team believed that it was important that the patient have dignity and respect. He was a person in his own right who had plans developed with him and not for him. He was involved each step of the way. As an autonomous person, his choices were acknowledged and accepted.

Initially, the team and the patient were working toward achieving the patient's optimum level of functioning. Ultimately, it was the patient who chose to abandon this goal. Working with Patrick was gratifying because he was open and honest with himself and with the providers when he made his decision about his life choices. It was a decision he made knowing what the outcome would be.

Nurses and other medical professionals recognize that many factors have an influence on health. Determinants of health are the broad range of personal, social, economic, and environmental factors that determine individual and population health. In Patrick's past and present situation, these factors no doubt helped shape the choices available to him and the choices he made along the way.

MARIAN FACCIOLO

It Is My Life
Deirdre's Story

As an advanced practice nursing student, I met Carl, a man who was an in-patient at the agency where I did my practicum. Carl survived an initial trauma through the aggressive and expert care of acute medicine. However, he believed that he had been neglected throughout his recovery and adaptation to disability, because rehabilitation and continuing care were concerned with curing his body. Carl contended that by concentrating on curing, the hospital demonstrated a lack of interest in assisting him to "get on with life." Carl's story represents his journey from independence to a new reality that, in his words, "fosters dependence on the hospital."

Five years earlier, Carl had retired from an executive position. He and his wife moved to our area from the large metropolis where they had lived most of their married lives. They built a house on a nearby lake and looked forward to a peaceful retirement. Over the next two years, the marriage disintegrated, and the couple divorced.

Three years earlier, Carl had been driving home to his cottage when he experienced a severe motor vehicle accident. His car flipped over, and he was trapped inside, underwater. Witnesses to the accident managed to free him from the wreckage, but his heart had stopped beating. One of the witnesses was a physician; he performed CPR. Carl responded and was transported to the local acute care hospital, where he remained in a coma for eight weeks. When he awoke from the coma, he realized that he had spinal injuries that rendered his lower body immobile and limited his use of his right hand.

Eventually, he was transferred to the rehabilitation in-patient unit at my practicum agency. During his stay in rehabilitation, he developed decubitus ulcers, or bedsores, that were so severe he was transferred to the complex continuing care area of the same hospital. When I met him, he had five decubitus ulcers that were not healing.

Carl spoke of his perception that the hospital was not proactive in his care and accepted the fact that he was going to remain in hospital for a long time.

He stated that the physicians were no longer interested in him because he was chronic, and the process of healing was "taking too long." He expressed his opinion that the nurses were "more interested in who is going to coffee with whom" than in providing care. He cited errors in medication administration, refusal to follow a consistent protocol for dressing changes, and examples of the nursing routine taking priority over the patient's choices as evidence of his belief that the hospital lacked interest in his progress.

From the team's perspective, Carl was described as "non-compliant" and "difficult." He refused to follow a schedule of turning to alleviate pressure on his ulcers; he also frequently refused care, yelled at nurses, made demands for treatments not offered by the hospital, and searched the internet for "magical cures." The team expressed frustration but was genuinely concerned about Carl's recovery. They believed that he was unrealistic about the future and questioned his ability to make decisions based on their assumptions about brain damage that may have occurred at the time of the accident.

Here I was, a student in advanced practice nursing, trying to find a path that might help Carl and the team work together. This man's simple statement, "I am interested in living my life," provided me with direction. The challenge was to move away from the traditional nursing model, where nurses decide on what is realistic for the patient, to a model that would place Carl's wishes back at the centre of care. This was easier said than done.

Over time, I was able to negotiate a forum where Carl's wishes were heard. The team established a series of meetings that would be chaired by Carl. Here he could contribute as an equal member of the health care team.

I was disappointed that my practicum ended before Carl's first meeting could be arranged. I do not know how the meetings went or if Carl's life improved. I did learn a great deal about shifting the nursing perspective from one where nursing goals are the focus to one where the person is the centre of care.

It is often easier for us, as nurses, to see the patient as the problem. It is far more difficult to acknowledge that our way of nursing might be the problem.

Deirdre understood that the situation was complex and the relationships were not therapeutic. Carl had a lot of anger and resentment related to his belief that the choices he was making were not being respected. He was frustrated. The staff didn't believe Carl was working in partnership with them to achieve what they considered to be maximum health. They also wondered about a possible brain injury that could have affected Carl's quality of decision making. Deirdre recognized that Carl felt no one cared about what he wanted. She did well to bring the staff together with the patient to problem-solve. She advocated for a health care environment that is conducive to health and well-being. She made the patient the centre of care and set it up so he could have an integral part in moving forward.

DNR or No DNR?
Marian's Story

This is a story about Lunilla, an elderly Italian lady. We got the referral at our agency to provide palliative care in the home. Prior to coming to our area, the patient had been living in another city. She was being cared for by her family with the help of in- home services. Lunilla ended up in hospital after aspirating and subsequently developed aspiration pneumonia. She was treated at the hospital and discharged home.

Lunilla was a direct admission to our program. I set up a home visit to meet her and her family. Communication was at times difficult because of some language barriers. When I made the visit, it was obvious that the family was distraught. Lunilla was lying in bed. She had a G-tube in place, and bags hanging from an IV pole next to the bed. Urine was draining into a catheter bag hanging from the bed rail. Lunilla was unresponsive when she was spoken to. She was semi-comatose and unable to take anything by mouth. Her skin was breaking down. Her periodic moaning and facial expressions indicated to me that she was in pain. These symptoms were also noted during her stay in the hospital.

We received the referral from the hospital and initiated services, including nursing for wound care, G-tube feedings, foley catheter care, and palliative support. The occupational therapist was consulted for home safety and equipment. There was some support set up to help the patient/family with personal care and provide some respite. Like other semi- comatose patients, she needed to be turned and positioned regularly. She required complete care.

While she had been in the hospital, Lunilla was a "full code." This meant that if she stopped breathing, she would have to be resuscitated. The family was not prepared to let her go. They had power of attorney for personal care and were making the decisions for her. They believed she would want to be resuscitated. They did not want a do-not-resuscitate (DNR) order on her file. The family believed that Lunilla would choose this if she was able to communicate. The family also made it clear that they did not want her in a nursing home or in a residential hospice.

I felt that during my visit, a lot of ground was covered. I understood where the family members were coming from with their wishes. I struggled with the fact that they wanted to keep Lunilla alive at all costs. Was there a conflict of values here? I told myself that I needed to remain open, support them, and help them through the process. Lunilla was going to die eventually. The question was when, and what would she go through before reaching that end. They wanted her on a ventilator if it came to that.

The family told me they did not want their mom to get morphine, as they believed that she would not survive this medication. The family believed that its's use would cause further deterioration of her condition. I suggested they try extra strength Tylenol. This could be crushed and given through the G-tube. Before I left, I pointed to the signs of pain that Lunilla was exhibiting and suggested that they consider the use of a pain medication. As I left the house that day, the daughter walked with me to the door. She told me that she loved my blue eyes. My heart warmed as I knew it was her way of giving me her approval. They did start using the Tylenol regularly. One tablet turned to two, and then it was given at regular intervals. Lunilla did get some pain relief and her cries of pain diminished.

Lunilla was palliative, so it was important to have a doctor in the area to support her, the family, and nurses during her decline. The nurses would need to have a physician to provide orders for different medications as necessary, and to make a home visit if required. Our protocol in the community setting was to have this support for the patient when palliation was provided at home. Initially the family said no, they would take her to the ER rather than change the doctor who they trusted and spoke Italian. Unfortunately, their doctor did not live close to our area.

Over the following weeks, I worked closely with the family to get the personal support hours adjusted to suit their schedule. I worked closely with the nurses to broach the subject of DNR periodically. They eventually agreed to have a doctor in the area to oversee her care and manage her pain. I called the available doctor to provide preliminary information about the patient. I told him about the issues and how things had evolved. I explained how they had progressed in their thoughts about DNR. At first, they were adamant there would not be one. Later, they agreed to have one, but then, after further discussion, they changed their minds again. The doctor listened well and, in my view, had a good starting point and understanding of this family. He began his own relationship with them. This doctor was able to bring the family to understand exactly what was meant by a DNR and the implications for Lunilla. He was able to help them understand why it was needed to preserve their mom's dignity during her palliative care.

I believe that it was a team effort to support this patient/family throughout the dying process. The visiting nurse was in good communication with both the family and me. The family felt supported. The agency providing the personal support was able to provide continuity of care for the patient and family. The palliative care doctor was able to complete an integral part of the plan for this client to meet her death with dignity and to help the family come to terms with this important decision.

To decide to put a DNR in place can be a difficult one for many families and for some more than others. While providing care for this family, I reflected on what I knew about the Italian culture. I had been exposed to a lot of it because my husband is Italian. Italian people tend to be very supportive of their family and elders when they are sick and dying. Early in our marriage my husband had expressed his distaste for DNR. He indicated that he would feel like he would be responsible for the death of his parent and carry guilt for the rest of his life. Family is very important to them. They respect their elders and want only what they think is best for them. I reflected on my own values about pain control and DNR. Nurses work to assist patients and families to optimum levels of health and support during the palliative process. Pain control is one aspect that needs particular attention throughout palliation and end-of-life care. Assisting with a plan for end- of- life care and decision making is another one. I believe that in this instance, my values and the family's values were not in conflict. This family wanted to ensure their mother's preferences would be respected.

He Has Suffered Enough
Deirdre's Story

Adam was a thirty-six-year-old man who was born to a single mother in the late 1960s. He was premature and weighed only 2.2 pounds at birth. His mother gave him up for adoption. Somehow, without any family member pulling for him, he survived. He eventually was taken in by a foster family. Unfortunately, his disabilities proved too difficult for the foster family to manage, and he was placed in the care of an institution when he was five. His foster family maintained contact with him throughout his life. They had power of attorney for his medical care.

Adam experienced many severe disabilities. He was blind, had seizures, and had a profound developmental disability. He couldn't walk or talk. However, Adam had a joy in living that rivalled that of any non-disabled person.

I first met him when he was thirty. His body was very twisted. He lay on a wheelchair called a supine transporter. This was basically a bed on wheels. His left leg was bent upward toward his ear, and his right leg was permanently flexed. He could flail his arms and would wave them around while he let out an ear-piercing scream. It sounded like he was in pain, but this was his joyful sound. Despite all his disabilities, he won my heart. I looked forward to our time together. Caring for him was always a joy.

One day, Adam became very ill. He was rushed to the hospital. The doctor stated that he needed surgery, but because of Adam's physical condition, the physician was worried about his quality of life after surgery. The doctor stated that without the surgery, Adam would die. He believed that Adam had "suffered enough" and that the best course of action was to care for him as palliative. With heavy hearts, Adam's family agreed to place him on palliative care. Adam was unable to take anything by mouth, so he was given no food or fluid. He was kept comfortable, and his family stayed with him until his death.

I, however, was furious. I did not agree that Adam had "suffered enough." I did not believe that his life was one of suffering. I knew Adam as a person of great joy, who loved others and who many loved. How could his doctor and his family decide he had "suffered enough"?

I struggled with my personal feelings. I knew that, as a professional, I really had no standing in the decisions that were being made. Yet, my heart cried for Adam.

I knew that the foster family made this difficult decision with Adam's best interests in mind. Yet I could not agree that this decision was "best" for Adam.

After much reflection and angst, I decided that there was only one thing I could do for Adam. My decision was to be kind to his family and support them as Adam went through the process of dying. As much as I disagreed with the decision to make Adam palliative, I also realized that, as a professional RN, my role was to support Adam as he journeyed through life and death. His journey touched me deeply.

As I watched him die, I saw the fighting spirit in him continue. He engaged those of us around him the way he always had, with his ability to connect to us without words. Without words, he invited us into his world, his joy, his sorrow, his love for us.

Adam died seven days after he was declared palliative. I have often reflected on the lessons that I learned from him: lessons about connecting to others; listening and learning, despite my personal feelings; finding joy; supporting families.

I will never know if the family's decision was truly in Adam's "best interests." In the same circumstances, I might have made a different decision. Yet I do not know if my decision would have been "best" either. He was a young man with severe disabilities. He touched my heart in a way that no one else has.

Since his death, I have never again looked at "best interests" decision-making as a simple, obvious choice. Deciding what is "best" for others is not a matter for personal opinion. In Adam's case, the decision about what was "best" seemed so clear to me. Yet, as I look back, I ask myself how his physician and family could have such a different opinion.

Who is right? Who is wrong? What is best? Not easy questions. No easy answers.

My Brother Needs Help
Marian's Story

I was working as a case manager in the community when I did an assessment on Helen, a ninety-one-year-old lady who lived alone in a one-bedroom apartment. She was a lovely person, quiet, calm, and non-imposing. She was able to answer the questions and provide all the needed information for the assessment. Although she had some chronic medical conditions, she was able to function quite independently. Her main difficulty was that she was not safe to take a shower or a bath on her own. Because she was unsteady, she used a walker to get around. She was eligible for our program and was put on a waiting list for personal care. We had a long waiting list, and I did feel bad that I could not offer her in-home assistance right away. Her daughter lived about three and a half hours away and came every second weekend to help her with shopping and a bath. Helen gave me permission to phone her daughter to provide an update on the visit and explain why her mother would be on a waiting list.

At the time of my visit, Helen expressed concern for her ninety-three-year-old brother, who lived in the same building. She wondered if I could visit him to see if there was anything I could do for him. She was worried, as he had trouble getting around, cooking, shopping, doing laundry. I told her that I would need his consent to do this. She said that he had a family doctor, but had not seen him in many years. She told me that she would talk with her brother and get back to me.

All new referrals at our agency go through a central intake. At one time, several years before this, all referrals also needed to be done by a physician. This was no longer the case. Families and/or other professionals could make a referral. The patient would usually be aware of this and in agreement.

A few weeks after my visit to Helen, she called me to let me know that her brother, Bob, had agreed to have a home visit to be assessed. I called him and set up a visit for the next week. Bob was a tall, lanky man with thinning hair. He did not use a walker or cane in the apartment. I could tell he wasn't used to having visitors. He spent most of his time alone. I sensed a distrust. He told me that he hated doctors and had not seen one in many years.

He managed to get through the assessment. He was able to provide the information I required. I could tell he was a rather private person. It was not easy for him to share health and private details with a stranger. I had met other people like him before and understood his reluctance to share personal information. There was something about him that made me look a bit deeper. Something about Bob reminded me of my own father. This man was private, fiercely independent, and proud.

As time went on, it seemed to get a bit easier for him to talk to me. He was able to give general information about his health status and other issues. When talking about his health and function, he told me that it was quite difficult for him to get around now. It was difficult because of his legs. After telling me this, he took off his slippers and socks and rolled up his pants. I could hardly believe what I saw. Both feet and lower legs were very mottled, somewhat lumpy and bluish gray with red spots. The colour improved at his knees. I had seen people with circulatory problems before, and toes that were gangrenous, but never such a wide-spread condition. I knew it was not good.

I told him that I was concerned about his legs and that I thought he needed to go to the hospital. The look on his face told me he already knew the situation was grave. He was looking to me to tell him that he was fine, and that everything would be fine. He did not want to go to hospital. I asked him if he would at least go to see his family doctor. He told me that he would think about our conversation. He would sleep on it. I told him that I would call him the next day to see what he decided. I left him and called his doctor to tell him what I had found at my visit and the plan.

The next day when I called, Bob agreed to go to the emergency department. I called ahead and spoke with the nurse in charge to let her know the situation.

Bob never came out of the hospital. He died not long after his admission.

Bob was afraid of what was happening to him. He needed to know that no one would force him to do anything he did not want to do. I believe that we developed good rapport during my time with him, and he came to trust me. He seemed to know that I wanted the best for him and that whatever choice he made would be respected.

Ethical Distress
Marian's Story

I was working as a case manager in the community. The workload was getting progressively heavier. Computer assessments took more time to complete, and the acuity and complexity of patient care was increasing. The agency was trying different models of care to see what might work best. In a span of several years, the model was changed a few times. A friend of mine was aware of the changes and likened it to "shuffling chairs on the *Titanic*." This analogy made sense at the time.

The problem was that the workload was very heavy. As well, case managers were expected to meet standards such as frequency of visits, response times for charting, and phone calls etc. The case manager was expected to be out in the field with the patients and families to do assessments, reassessments, and plan adjustments. It was important to share information, plan care, link to other community resources, and help the patient/family navigate the system. Documentation was a key part of the job. It was important to check phone messages several times a day. It was not unusual for some caseloads to have as many as twenty messages a day. The messages needed to be listened to, prioritized with follow up. Our message machine informed the caller that a callback could be expected by the end of the next business day. Given those heavy caseloads, this standard was often unable to be met. Nurses would try constantly to deal with the workload demands, and some would go to the person in charge to notify them of the issue. Most often, the person in charge was sympathetic but seemed unable to do much about it.

Many of the nurses worked unpaid overtime hours to get the job done, since it was difficult to get overtime hours approved. Some staff felt embarrassed that they could not do all the necessary work within the allotted time.

The agency had a process to flag workload issues. It included the completion of a "Professional Responsibility Form." Completion of the form required details to indicate specific situations and indications of the risks to justify more support for the case manager. A few case managers at our agency had done this. These forms were being completed in other areas of the province as well to signal that there was a significant concern regarding caseloads.

I completed one of these forms. It happened at a time when a few other nurses/case managers had also completed them. A meeting was arranged with a representative of the human resource team and management. It felt good to have others there who shared the same concerns. I was able to hear the issues reported by others, which were like my own. As a group, we felt more empowered to express our views. I was able to make a case for the potential risks to my patients if things continued as they were.

I realized this was not an issue about me or the other nurses around me who were willing to speak up and ask for change. Case managers were under a lot of stress and working in a culture some considered not conducive to open dialogue. At the time, it was my view that there was not enough staff to do what was required to properly care for all our patients and their families. At the time, I described it as "ethical distress." This label gave me comfort to express openly my obligation to my patients and their families to provide the care in a timely fashion. I believed that the safety of my patients could be at risk if time did not allow me to provide the proper care and follow up.

Although it was beyond my control to change the situation, I could at least try by assertively going through the formalized process. At a minimum the College of Nurses would expect this course of action.

Initially, the result of the joint meeting of staff, management, and HR was empowerment for staff. Some nurses who were timid or uncomfortable about speaking were able to hear what others had to say. They realized they were not alone and, gradually, they felt more at ease about speaking up as everyone was having the same issue, which required resolution. The meeting had a positive outcome for me and one other nurse, as it led to a reduction in our case numbers. We were still busy, but our schedules were not quite as bad and the level of risk within our caseloads was mitigated.

To my knowledge, when there was an issue and the "Professional Responsibility Form" was submitted in the future, the agency did not bring nurses together to discuss it and problem solve. Instead, they held individual meetings with the nurse who had filled out the form.

Our group had requested that patient caseload numbers be reduced so risks could be mitigated and expectations for follow-up time could be met. If this was not an option, we asked that the message on the machine be changed to reflect our reality. It was suggested that many of the messages left on the answering machine did not need to be addressed quickly, as we were not working in the acute setting (that is, we weren't in a hospital), where things were more urgent and often a matter of life and death. Meanwhile, over the years, the acuity and complexity of patients and situations in the community increased significantly.

Even after having an open dialogue to discuss the problems, the issue was not adequately resolved. Changing the phone message was not considered an option. The agency rarely approved overtime. It was my impression that the agency needed us to do more with less.

In my view, the process and end results served to frustrate and demoralize the case managers and built a culture in which nurses felt powerless and unsupported. Did the agency lack the power and/or the resources to produce change? The notion of "ethical distress" continued to fester because the issues were not adequately resolved, and some staff members felt that they were not really listened to or respected. Some came away questioning whether management understood the real life and circumstances of the case managers out in the field.

In situations where the demands of the job impact negatively on care, it is important that nurses strongly advocate for change. Nurses are expected to care for patients, but there are limits to what they can do, especially when they work in a system that espouses caring but is frequently driven by economics. Although it is necessary to consider the economics of the health care system, I believe this needs to be balanced with the needs of the patients. Also, it is not unreasonable to expect that staff workload align with what is manageable. In addition, it is not unreasonable to provide an environment whereby staff feel their voices are heard, respected, and valued.

12. Repairs and Maintenance

As individuals, we tend to continually look at our lives and try to figure out what is working and what isn't working. What makes us happy? What is causing us unhealthy stress? What areas are out of balance? Where are the gaps? How are we coping and what needs to change for us to be in better balance?

For nurses, the demands of work can be huge. Sometimes the demands are related to workload or hours of work or the complexity and/or acuity of the patient population. They may stem from the many risk situations (physical, emotional, mental) we encounter for the patients, their families, or ourselves. Sometimes, they boil down to a lack of support from the health care system that we serve. In order to avoid the effects of chronic stress, burnout, and PTSD, nurses need to continually evaluate the work situation, just as they continually evaluate their own health and safety.

Nurses tend to go into the profession for the right reasons. As nurses get more experience, they can bring more to the work they do. They can take an active role in identifying issues of concern and offer their suggestions for solutions and improvements for daily and ongoing concerns. The outcome will inevitably be improved health of individual nurses, their longevity in the profession, and ultimately a more rewarding career.

Nurses do not necessarily have full control of the environment they work in. Therefore, it is also incumbent on the employer to put in place supports that will help bring the nurse back to health if the stressors become too heavy to bear. Stories by nurses highlight the effects on the nurse when the necessary supports are present and when they are not.

In this chapter, we can see some of the critical issues faced by the nurses who shared their stories and bared their souls. You can feel the depth of despair experienced by these nurses. One nurse shows what happens when trauma is not acknowledged and there is no support from the system. At a minimum, nurses need to have support to maintain themselves within the profession over time. They also need support to repair damages that have been done.

Other stories show the value of quality leadership, enlightened management, teamwork, public support, and paying it forward. They demonstrate how leadership can foster growth and development, empowering and encouraging nurses to excel.

At the end of this chapter, I have included three stories about COVID-19. Prior to the COVID-19 pandemic, there were issues related to nursing that needed to be addressed. Many of these are visible in the nursing stories from the front line. With the onset of the pandemic, a spotlight has been shone on nursing, the role of nurses and the environment they presently work in. The COVID stories included here are honest, heartfelt and insightful. They highlight some of the shortcomings of an already ailing system that have been further exacerbated by the demands of a health emergency. Stress, workload, risks, and burnout are just a few of the things that will need to be addressed to repair, maintain and sustain the system and the nurses working in it. A recurrent theme in nursing is that nurses often feel undervalued for the work they do. I think that we, as nurses, need to ask ourselves as a group if we contribute to this by either our unwillingness or inability to speak up about the value of the work we do. If nurses themselves don't speak up to promote the value of their work, it may very well be interpreted as nurses themselves minimizing the value of the work they do.

The nurse needs to engage and understand the patient in order to provide empathy. Being invested like this can be a risk to the nurse. However, if the nurse is detached, the patient may not feel that the nurse cares. The relationship will not facilitate healing. If the nurse gets too attached, there is the potential for tremendous stress and burnout. It is critical that a balance be reached both for the protection of the nurse and the healing process of the patient.

I believe that stress and burnout can be mitigated by a working environment that supports the nurse. When I look back, I am amazed at the things I could endure or overcome at work when the support was there from my direct supervisor or manager. Concurrently, the culture of the nurses' working environment can be such that nurses not only survive but also grow and flourish.

A "grow and flourish" culture would go a long way to improve the system that is presently in place. Taking good care of nurses will result in maximizing care for patients.

A theme of many of the stories in this book is that nurses need to listen to and "be with" the patient. This will lead to better results. This theme also needs to be applied for nurses. We should tell the system what supports we require as we care for people. If the system listens, patients will benefit because there will be healthier nurses.

Children in the Emergency Department
Jennifer's Story

I met with Jennifer, who shared a few nursing stories from her time spent in the emergency department of a busy hospital.

We received a call from the paramedics' line to alert us at the emergency (ER) department that they were sending us a baby in distress. We assembled the team in our pediatric room. The baby, born at home to a teenage mother, arrived at the ER department. It was an unwanted pregnancy. The teenager had tried to hide the pregnancy from family and friends and was quite successful at doing so.

She ended up giving birth at home after she locked herself in the bathroom. The parents knew something was wrong and tried to get into the bathroom. In order to hide or muffle the sounds and cries of the baby, she tried to drown the baby in the toilet. This didn't work. It was terrible.

The baby was still alive when she was taken to hospital and when we met her. She still had a pulse. The pediatric team was ready for her when she arrived. There was still a pulse, but it was too low. We got an intravenous going and tried everything we could to save her. We were not able to keep the baby alive. We lost her. We were unsuccessful.

The mom had come through the ER on a stretcher and was taken to the labour and delivery (L and R) unit. We never met her. She had a retained placenta and went directly to L and R to have the contents removed. After the baby passed away, we were told that while in L and R, the mom claimed she was never pregnant and there was no baby. She was in complete denial.

When this happened, I was a young nurse in my early twenties. I had been working in ER for only a couple of years. It was tough. It was really tough. I didn't have any kids at the time. It bothered me. It was difficult, but I don't think I would have done as well with it had I been where I am now, with my kids. This happened and we went back to work and finished our shift. We worked twelve-hour shifts, so we needed to finish our shift and deal with the next trauma coming in. I had to finish my shift and go back to work the next day. It was traumatic and stressful.

I am glad I worked in ER when I did, even though there was a lot of death, trauma, and abuse with kids. I don't think I would have been able to do it for as long as I did if I had kids of my own. I worked about six years in total in ER departments.

We did have one debrief session. It was a couple of weeks after the event happened. I don't think it helped that much. The paramedics who had to deal with it were pulled off the road that day. The trauma was deemed such that they needed to cope with it before going back to work.

There was another situation of child abuse. A two-year-old South Asian girl was brought to the ER with submersion burns. This happens when a child is put in water that is too hot and they end up with burns to the skin. I had been told that there is a cultural practice that may have been used by the parents to control their children when they are misbehaving. Her dad brought her in to ER because she would not stop crying. There was a language barrier with this family. When we examined her, we found that her skin was extremely red and blistered from the waist down. She had been scalded. The police were called and there was an investigation.

Another situation that I recall was with a young child between eighteen and twenty-four months old. The child was brought into the ER by the grandmother. She was beside herself. The child was in extreme pain. The parents were teenagers and were separated. Each teenager lived with their respective parents and shared custody of the child. At the time of the incident, the child was staying with the biological dad. The dad had gone out and had arranged for his mother to babysit the child.

Every time the grandmother tried to move the baby's arm, the baby screamed. We did an examination, assessment, and X-rays. The baby was found to have multiple fractures throughout the body. Babies don't have fractures the same way as adults. They are called greenstick fractures. This baby was found to have fractures in different stages of healing. We had a team of specialists come to our hospital to take over the case. A criminal investigation for child abuse was initiated.

We made the baby comfortable. He was transferred to the floor for admission. Unfortunately, we often don't get the follow-up information. The child protection agency was brought in. We did not get a whole lot of information other than that.

There was a multiple-vehicle car accident. The victims came to our hospital. There was a minivan, which crashed with another vehicle and flipped several times. There were two families involved and they all came into our ER department on backboards with collars. There was a young baby in one of the vehicles. The paramedics had to tell the mother that the baby had been crushed and unable to survive.

I have to say that throughout my career, working for six years in ER, there was only the one time that there was a debriefing—and that, as I mentioned, was a couple of weeks after the incident. They wonder why nurses go on stress leave.

It was at this point that Jennifer started to cry. It was a sad, unexpected overflow of tears. She allowed herself a moment to recall her own feeling of grief. I felt her sadness and couldn't help but shed a few of my own tears. I wasn't even there for these incidents, but I had enough of my own sad experiences that I could totally relate. Jennifer took hold of herself. She told me that the paramedics saw more flesh in one of the vehicles. They looked closer and found what they thought at first was an elbow. It wasn't an elbow. As it turned out, it was the baby's head, crushed and unrecognizable.

Jennifer did not get the support she required. When I spoke with her, I was reminded that nurses are exposed to traumatic events and emotionally draining situations. In order to remain effective and avoid burnout, a nurse needs support from the working environment. Nurses also need to personally find ways to replenish.

Shared Knowledge of Leadership
Sharon M.'s Story

Sharon's story relates a better way to deal with this kind of work and is a good contrast to Jennifer's story.

After graduating from nursing, I applied to do outpost nursing and was accepted. I never ended up doing it. Through a bizarre set of circumstances, I ended up instead getting a job at the Montreal Children's Hospital. It was my ideal position: a pediatric emergency nurse.

During orientation, my manager informed me that emergency nursing is not what you see on television. She said it was not all blood and gore, as most people think. Unfortunately, my first three days in ER were an "orientation by fire." Each of those three days brought in another child who had been involved in a motor vehicle accident. All three of those children died from their injuries.

Fortunately, my manager was amazing and called me to her office to debrief me. Of course, I was distraught. This would have been difficult for even a seasoned nurse. My manager was tuned in to what I was going through. She noticed that I looked overwhelmed and upset. She brought me into her office, and we talked. She talked about her own past struggles having to deal with trauma. She too was feeling it this day. She talked about the fact that these were normal feelings.

Because of this debrief, I was better able to move forward. She saw me, she cared about me, and she acted upon it. She told me that her door was open, and I could come to talk with her at any time if I needed to do so.

This was a lesson that I carried with me to all the emergency departments where I worked. Whenever I was in charge and there was a critical incident, a death, or trauma, I would ask the "team" involved to take a few minutes to debrief. I would ask them to get out of the emergency department, go for a coffee, or get some fresh air. They would go out in a group of two or three and commiserate about the event. They would come back to the unit better able to face the next patient. Often, the next patient might be something mundane, so there could be some time to do this.

I can remember being in charge when a child with cancer came in and was bleeding. The hematology-oncology MD was frantic to get blood infused. It was a crisis. By the time it was hooked up, the child had passed away. The doctor kept telling the parents that she was sorry. She was obviously upset and started to cry. She rushed out of the trauma room and ran to the bathroom. I followed her there. She was overcome with grief, sadness, and frustration. She was sobbing uncontrollably. She didn't want the parents to see that she was crying. I remembered my very wise manager telling me that crying was okay in front of parents. It shows that you obviously care that you are affected by this child's death—it is a normal reaction to a life cut too short. And my manager said to never apologize for crying. That is not to say that a nurse will cry for every patient, but for whatever reason, some affect you more than others.

Sharon recognizes the value of debriefing and is appreciative of her manager, who understood what she was going through. She had a good role model. At the start of her time in that ER, her trauma was noticed, and she was supported through it. Sharon was lucky to have someone who understood.

Later on in her career, she tried to create a work environment where traumatic experiences were acknowledged and nurses received support through those difficult experiences. Sharon did well to "pay it forward" to the physician and other nurses.

As health care workers, we need to have the supports in place to take care of us so we can continue to care for others. Today, many workplaces have employee assistance programs, but this does not negate the need for more immediate supports, such as debriefing sessions and a supportive work environment.

A Night Shift to Remember
Mary's Story

This case went wrong right from the start. I was working for a private agency. I had been scheduled to do a night shift for an elderly lady with cancer. She previously had received chemotherapy and consequently lost all her hair. She was end-stage. Her husband and their neighbour were the main caregivers. The agency called me to provide the details of the patient's condition and the home address.

Whenever I worked the night shift, I had the habit of driving to the house before my shift began. This way, I would not be searching in the dark. That night, at ten forty-five p.m., I knocked at the door of the house where my patient was supposed to reside. It was in total darkness. I heard a deep loud bark within the house. A very large man answered the door in his underwear. He was holding the collar of a big, muscular bulldog. He was not impressed that I had awakened him. It was the wrong house. I apologized profusely. He turned around and slammed the door in my face. There was no such thing as a cellphone back then. I drove around to find a phone booth.

Finally, I found a phone booth and called my agency.

"Oops, my mistake. Did I say 506? I meant 509. Three doors down."

Now I was half an hour late. Me, who is never late. I was also quite upset.

I arrived at my patient's home to find that my patient's husband was furious. I can't blame him. He was exhausted caring for his wife, and he just wanted to go to bed. A quick report from him and he was off to bed.

His wife was palliative, and I was the first night nurse to do a shift. Shift nursing was arranged to give him some much-needed relief. I proceeded to do positioning, skin care, mouth care, and catheter care. Every four hours, she had injections for pain. During the days and evenings, the neighbour, who was a nurse, was able to help with the medication administration. There was a communication book in place. It indicated the times and dosage of pain medication. There was no mention of any confusion or aggression.

I recall that the patient was very thin and fragile. When I spoke with her, she only answered yes or no. I spoke to her quietly to offer a drink, back care, or medication. She did not seem confused, just weak.

Her bedroom was small and very cluttered. It was loaded with furniture. The chair I sat in had been squeezed into the corner of the room. It was difficult to navigate around the room. I was frustrated that the person who did the initial home visit did not get the family to arrange the room so that one could move around without tripping or getting lodged between two pieces of furniture. It should have been set up better to facilitate function.

At five a.m., the patient woke up, very confused. She had received the pain medication about an hour and a half before waking up. Now she was trying to get out of bed. She was very restless, and I thought I could help her change position so I could rub her back. She wanted to sit up, so I helped her into a sitting position and started to rub her back.

She got agitated, pushed me, and then wrestled me to the floor between the dresser and bed. I shouted out several times, calling for her husband to help. He did not answer. She was all over me and would not let me up! For a frail person, she seemed very strong. I couldn't get through or reason with her. My main objective was to keep her safe. It all happened so quickly. I did not have a chance to brace myself. Finally, she tired herself out. I was able to get her back to bed.

She did not get hurt at all, but the pain in my back was horrible. I waited until seven a.m., when her husband got up, to tell him what happened. He said he did not hear a thing. He told me he had taken his hearing aids out and slept on his good ear.

After I left the house, I went to the hospital. I was examined and found to have four torn muscles in my back. I was in a bad state. You could see the muscles "twitching" on my back. My employer was notified, and I was off work for six months. I needed physiotherapy for three months. Surprisingly, my patient passed away two days after the incident. It was amazing how strong she was. I never worked another night shift in a home!

I had never had such a thing happen to me before. I had worked in the hospital for years. While in the community, I had worked a lot of night shifts in homes. I was angry at the agency and the person in charge who set up the visit. It was a private agency and I did not have a high regard for the owner. They had given me the wrong address, which subsequently made me late and the husband angry. It started things off on the wrong foot. I completed an incident report. My injury was so bad that I ended up on Workman's Compensation for six months. Still to this day, when I reach to clean windows or wash a floor on my hands and knees, my back muscles hurt.

I don't recall any support from the agency. I never got a call to discuss it or how I was doing. When I recovered, I went back to the agency. I did one day shift. After that I moved on to a pediatric agency. It was not long afterward that I decided to take an early retirement. I felt broken.

The stories from Jennifer and Mary speak to the historical minimization of the effects of stress and trauma on nurses. They also speak to the ethical distress nurses feel when they are unable to meet the standards of care and address risks when they need to do so. Until very recently, nurses were expected to deal with traumatic experiences without any assistance. In telling of her experiences in the ER, Jennifer indicates that debriefing was just an afterthought two weeks after an incident. There was no consideration that Jennifer's trauma could have had serious psychological consequences.

Sharon worked in three different ER departments over her many years in nursing. She reported to me that one debriefing was so worthwhile for her that she found a way to pay it forward to her staff when she was in charge. However, during her many years of nursing with traumatic events and deaths, there was never any formal type of debriefing sessions. Mary received no support from the agency where she worked after her trauma. The impact on her was debilitating and eventually resulted in early retirement.

Running on Fumes
Rita's Story

I now work for an agency that helps transition people from home or a retirement home into a nursing home. The people I work with are cognitively impaired and have significant behavioural issues. I see them when they have their name on a waiting list for placement. They are very high on the list because of their living situation and the inability of family or staff to manage them any longer. They are usually on a crisis list for placement. My job is to get to know them, their behaviours and their family. Then I can better help them adjust to going into a nursing home. I establish rapport and provide support prior to the move. Once they do go to the nursing home, I provide some continuity for them while they are there initially.

Prior to this job, I worked as a nurse in a nursing home. I did this for eight years. I worked full-time on an Alzheimer's/dementia floor with thirty-two patients. There were other units in the nursing home, but my unit had the people with behavioural problems. I worked the day shift and had four personal support workers who I oversaw. I was in charge. This entailed doing admissions, discharges, calling the physicians when needed, addressing issues of concern, and giving out the medications. The medications included the individual ones and the as-needed (PRN) ones.

Working in this area had many challenges and many wonderful small moments. Things got very difficult when there were three behavioural patients on the unit at the same time. These residents could be very aggressive and demanded a lot of time. Sometimes, they could be violent. I found it more difficult with the men, as they were stronger. When patients were violent, we would refer them for a psychogeriatric consult and make a referral to the behavioural support team. The waiting list for admission for a specialized assessment was very long. In the meantime, we had to try to deal with the behaviours in the home. There were PRN medication orders, but often this was not enough to manage the situation.

These patients can be so cognitively impaired that they don't understand what they are saying or doing at all. I have been kicked, sworn at, hit, and once swatted on my back so hard I thought I would pass out. This is a recipe for disaster. Sometimes, it would get so bad that we had to send the person to the acute care hospital to be seen and treated there. The hospital stay time can vary. In the hospital, they have a reassessment and usually have their medications adjusted. They come back a bit better able to be managed.

This was most likely to happen to those patients whose behaviour was so challenging that they were waiting to go to Waypoint, the local psychiatric hospital. This is a specialized unit where, after admission, the person will have a thorough examination, a review of medications and medical conditions, relevant tests, and review of behaviours. The patient will be seen by specialists, and recommendations will be made. Patients often end up staying there for months in order to ensure safety and best function on return to the nursing home.

All this contributed to a high level of stress. One never knew what situation one was going to walk into each day. There were many challenges, and as a nurse working in the nursing home, you found ways to deal with them. I found there was a high rate of sick calls by staff. When it is so stressful, it is difficult for staff to keep coming to work each day. It was difficult to find someone to replace a sick staff member, so most often when someone was off sick, you found yourself short-staffed. Being short-staffed was an ongoing issue.

The administration of medications is a major issue. Where I worked, we had blister packs and computerized pharmacy. As a nurse, you must find the best way to ensure your patient gets the medication. You look at what to put the medications into so the patient will swallow them. I never would leave medications by the bedside. It isn't safe to do so. Very often, I had to go back again and again.

If patients don't take their medications, there is an issue with dosing. It can affect when the next one should be given. At one time there was a sign on the medication cart: "DO NOT DISTURB THE NURSE while passing out medications." That was short-lived. The busiest time for medication pass is the morning and then again at bedtime. Pass is very busy. When it is busy and you are trying to pass out medications, there are constant interruptions by patients. This leads to medication errors. I can honestly say that most medication errors are due to high workload. I have had my share of them. Usually, it has been an issue of double dosing, rather than giving the wrong medication. Whenever there is a medication error, the nurse has the responsibility to complete a report on it. The other thing about medications is that if the patient doesn't take their medication, they can get aggressive. This leads to more problems, and even a simple thing such as bathing becomes more difficult.

Approach is key in dealing effectively with cognitively impaired and behavioural patients. They seem to sense when you are having a bad day. You could be having a bad day for any reason. Being understaffed is just one of them. If you are having one of these days, the patients know it. They read it, feel it, and hear it in you! They can feel you are rushed and stressed. They just seem to pick it up. You must check yourself at the door. The patients know by the tone of your voice that you are in a hurry. Sometimes the patients just want a few minutes of your undivided attention. If I had more staff to be there with the patients, I would not have needed to use nearly as many PRN medications as I did.

I would have liked to use a non-medical approach to manage patients. I have used it and it does work. The problem is that it takes more time, but it does work. It means you or the personal support worker (PSW) need to talk with the person one to one; walk with them in the halls; ask them if they want a drink and, if they do, get them one; ask if they need to go to the bathroom and, if they do, then go with them and help them.

Another issue is that patients are at risk for falls. This can be because of the use of PRN medications, which can increase the falls risk. We have patients who try to climb out of bed or abandon their walkers. To help us manage risks we have bed alarms, chair alarms, and floor mats. Patients are only allowed to have seat belts used on a wheelchair if they can undo them. Otherwise they are seen as restraints, and that is not to be done. Patients still fall and then get fractures. If a seat belt is used on a wheelchair, the person needs to be checked hourly, and it needs to be documented hourly and every shift.

We also take care of patients who decline and become palliative. They usually require more care and attention when this happens. There are no provisions to have extra staff when a patient becomes palliative, even though they need more care.

There are annual and semi-annual reports to do, and policies and procedures to follow. The RAI [resident assessment instrument] computerized assessment is part of it. I am a registered practical nurse (RPN). At one point, I felt that my skill level wasn't enough, as I was very overwhelmed at work. It is also hard to do everything right when you are running. Yes, I got an orientation, but in the real world, when I had to take charge of the unit, it was different. I could call the charge nurse if needed. She oversaw all the different units in the nursing home. I often found that the charge nurse, who was an RN, did not have enough experience. Often, they were new graduates.

I believe funds are limited in the long-term care system and nursing homes. Meanwhile, the people working there need more orientation and mentoring. They need to learn about what to report and how to deal with behaviours. These specific strategies to deal with behaviours are not things you learn when you take your nursing certificate. There is training in non-violent intervention, although I did not get it before working in a nursing home. I believe it should be mandatory and taught before you get thrown into the job. Everyone needs behavioural training and education before working in a nursing home. This includes all the PSWs and nurses. We need training in how to approach people with dementia. We need training on how to give medications to people with dementia. I believe we also need a team of behavioural specialists who can help us work with people with behaviours. It would serve patients and staff well. We are all so busy running! We don't have the time to see, reflect, and do the planning required for our people.

There need to be more meetings in which we talk about high-risk patients. We need team conferences so we can share information, connect with each other as a group, and reflect about what worked and what did not with patients. These were few and far between. I can remember one of these meetings where we discussed a particular resident. This then led to looking at the number of times he had received a PRN medication for pain. We were stunned by the amount of pain medication he was getting. We decided that pain management was an issue, and we moved forward to solve this issue.

In many ways, I loved working with the geriatric population and the cognitively impaired. It was just that I got completely burned out. I knew it. I was never out on time. At times, I gave patients the extra attention they needed. I was then left charting late at the end of my shift. I think I cared too much. I needed to step back and take a good look at what was happening. I was getting impatient and grouchy. I was becoming increasingly unwell. My physical state was really suffering. My blood pressure was elevated. The workload was insane. Some nurses did not get involved with the patients and they got out on time. I got very tired and was so unhappy. Mostly, I found myself feeling very negative and bitchy at work with management. I got increasingly angry when things got worse and the sick calls by the PSWs were higher. I never heard from management unless there was a problem. I certainly did not feel valued or in any way appreciated in my job. Basically, there was too much work and not enough workers. There was very little respect for the work we did each day.

After a lot of thought, I left for a couple of months and took time for myself. I tried a couple of other nursing homes. I found that the problems were the same there. I think it isn't just the nurses that need more help but also the personal support workers. It was an impossible task to get everything done that was needed. I desperately wanted and needed a change. I just could not do it anymore and had to leave in order to save myself. I left the job in 2018.

Rita is very emotional as she tells her story about her work situation. In the recording that she made for this book, her frustration is evident when she speaks about her work. She was breaking down both physically and emotionally. Rita is sad, and she feels that she was working in an environment where she was powerless and not valued. She speaks about the lack of support with the day-to-day workload. There is never enough staff to support the people she needs to support each day. At some point after working in this environment, Rita gives up. She realizes that she has no voice. She feels she is not seen or heard and does not want this in her future.

Rita has ideas that could be instrumental in improving the quality of life and environment for the patients and staff. Perhaps it is time to ask the nurses and other front-line staff how they think the patients and their families can be better served. They know what they need to improve their working environments so they can do their jobs more effectively.

I Found My Voice
Nancy's Story

It was during the Mike Harris years in Ontario [1995 to 2002, when Mike Harris was premier of a Progressive Conservative provincial government] and nurses were being laid off. I had graduated in 1993 from Queen's University with my bachelor of science degree in nursing. I was excited about my chosen profession. I believed nursing was a profession to be respected. I was looking forward to my new role and thrilled to be embarking on this journey. I had a vision of what nursing would be like once I graduated. I thought nursing was a noble profession and I was anxious to get more hands-on experience. I had only been graduated for about a year and a half.

Because of the cutbacks in Ontario, I ended up with a new position on a cardiac unit in Montreal. It was on this unit that I met a cardiac surgeon who changed my perception and shocked me into action.

I was the charge nurse that morning. As was the routine, I did patient rounds with the physician covering that morning. We saw a few patients. Then, after attending to one of the patients with the physician, I asked the physician a question in front of the patient. As I recall, it was not anything that was inappropriate in my mind. The physician did not answer, but instead looked really upset. We went out into the hallway, and he started to yell and scream at me. He did not approve of being asked a question.

I was not the first nurse to experience his wrath. He was in the habit of acting like this on many occasions with different nurses. It was as if he questioned the nurse's right to be on an equal footing with him. The way he acted with me that day, I had seen him behave that way with other nurses.

I decided that he was a bully and I was not going to take it. He seemed to think it was all right for him to be loud, condescending, and disrespectful of the nurses. That day, I spoke up for myself. I raised my voice and told him what I thought of his loud, abusive behaviour. I let him know that it was appropriate for me to initiate a discussion about an issue. It could even be healthy. I told him I'd had enough of his ignorant and aggressive behaviour, and I would not have it any longer. I saw how he treated other nurses who were members of the team. He was taken aback. I don't think anyone had ever stood up to him before this.

My response to him must have stimulated some reflection on his part. After this encounter, I never witnessed him act that way with the nurses. The dynamic changed.

My experience working in the acute care setting and dealing with the hierarchy and bureaucracy that existed was difficult for me. It was not that long afterward that I left that hospital. Once I left, it was a good twenty-five years before I returned from the community to the acute care setting. In retrospect, I think nurses get more confident as we get more experience. We find our voices with experience and increased confidence in our abilities.

Nancy is honest about the work situation in the hospital. She recounts an event that many nurses at that time would not be surprised about. Although the environment and culture was hierarchical, most physicians were respectful and appreciative of their nursing colleagues. However, it was important for Nancy to speak up and challenge the doctor's behaviour.

MARIAN FACCIOLO

Community Leader in the Early 1990s
Marian's Story

Our leader, the executive director (ED), was relatively new to the organization. It was a community agency, and she was now at the helm. The previous leader had retired.

The new leader had regular "all staff" meetings to update everyone on what was happening within the agency and on new developments in the health care system that impacted our agency. She was open in her communication. She welcomed questions. She did her best to provide answers to staff. She referred to herself as a "participatory" leader. Looking back, in my view, she was much more than that.

At that time, there was a high need for people to have homemaking provided. This was not something the system offered then. It was deemed to be a needed service that required development. There were five different geographical boundaries in our area. In order to develop the new "Homemaking Only Program," she recruited four nurse case managers and one assistant. There was a representative from each of the geographic areas. I was one of the people chosen to develop the program. The parameters of the program were set out by the strategic planning committee that she had already established.

We met as a group regularly each week. While we met, our caseloads were covered so we did not have to continually play catch-up. We developed the policies and procedures for the program. Eligibility guidelines were developed as well as a flow chart. The program was incorporated into the patient assessment tool that we already had in place. As we developed the program, each of the group members went back to their respective case manager and support staff groups. We requested and got feedback about the planning and development. Although we had ideas, we were open to what our peers had to offer and took their ideas into consideration. It did not mean that all ideas could be used, but all were at least considered. We wanted the best possible outcome for the project and our patients. Our progress was reported to the ED and the strategic planning committee.

Once the program was developed, it needed to be disseminated. We put together a staff in-service to teach our peers and others about the new program. This included a review of the new chart, eligibility, and structure and prosess of the program. It also included a request for feedback on our own staff in-service. In order to ensure consistency with the use of the program and identify areas of concern, a committee was put together to review the new referrals regularly. There were representatives from each of the geographical areas on this committee. They examined files to review the patient's strengths and limitations, eligibility, and amount of time allotted. They also looked at levels of consistency between nurse case managers. This service review was done to ensure consistency in utilization and resource management. I was on the committee for a while, then someone else had a turn. Initially, it was important for staff with intimate knowledge of the program design to be involved.

There was great satisfaction when this project was completed. The nurses/case managers using the program were involved throughout. The nurses gave lots of input. We saw the program develop from start to finish. It was a quality program. Eventually, over time, further changes were made. This program later became the foundation for the development of a personal support worker program. It was very empowering for me to be involved in the design and implementation of this program. I believe it was empowering to my co-workers to be involved and give significant input to the program. It showed that their input was valued. Nurses are very closely aligned with the patient and can be pivotal in the role they can play to identify gaps in the system and make recommendations for improvements and quality care.

I chose to tell this story of leadership because the manager had a very supportive approach. She listened to staff. She was a person of integrity and, above all, she trusted us to develop the program. It was not an autocratic, top-down approach. It was grassroots and it worked. She was not disappointed with the outcome. For me, it made a difference. My perception of real leadership was altered, and it became a reference point for all things labelled "leadership." I was later asked to be part of a committee called

"Involving the Community in Planning" with the public health unit. As a steering member of this committee, I was intent on applying the knowledge that I had gained from our executive director.

Workshop Experience
Marian's Story

It was the late 1990s and I was working as a case manager in the community. I was asked to be part of the Central East Case Management Workshop group. This committee met about four times a year to plan a one-day workshop for case managers in our area. I committed for a three-year term. Each year, roles were established within the group. People generally put their own names forward or were selected to be part of or to lead a function. There were different roles: evaluations, brochure development, speakers, chairperson, etc. Every member contributed to generate a presenter list as far as speakers were concerned. This was a situation where the people participating on the committee were staggered so that there was an overlap of case managers each year. This way, people with previous experience could be part of the committee.

The actual workshop always took place on a Saturday. A typical workshop day would include the introduction to the day, a keynote speaker, lunch, breakout sessions in the afternoon, and a wrap-up session at the end of day. Case managers signed up ahead of time for the smaller afternoon sessions. Nurses enrolled in sessions according to area of interest and what they most wanted to learn about. Sometimes, it was hard to choose. There were so many good topics.

One of the goals of the workshop was that the actual day would be educational and energizing. It was a chance to talk with case managers from different areas and commiserate about some of our common issues. We could also find out what others were doing that was progressive and how they might have approached different issues. It was a chance to network with our peers, get and give information, feel connected. Topics might be something like "Solution-Focused Communication," "Advocacy with the Elderly," "Documentation and Legalities." I remember having some fantastic speakers, including a nurse/lawyer who spoke on the topic "Advocacy for the Elderly." The main thing was that the topics needed to be relevant. Some were repeated more than once over the years, but mostly topics varied and were meant to help us learn, become better at our jobs, and improve and expand our viewpoint.

Several case managers participated on the workshop planning committee. Each nurse case manager represented a different geographical region. We had a manager from one of the areas who also attended. I believe this was to ensure we kept within the guidelines and within the financial limits. She was there to support and offer advice if needed. Each of the participating agencies paid the registration fee for their own case managers.

Planning for the workshop was work, but fun. We put our heads together and collaborated to organize and execute a meaningful workshop, where there was lots of learning and lots of fun and laughter.

For me, it was an invaluable experience. The first year, I worked on the evaluations. I volunteered for this. I thought it was less intimidating than some of the other roles. The second year, I worked on speakers. There was always a lot of discussion about speakers. We brought our thoughts about the most relevant and timely topics for case managers. We always had several speakers. My final year on the committee, I was chosen to be the chairperson.

In my year as chairperson, just over 400 case managers attended. I believe it was the best-attended workshop. Evaluations were fantastic, and it was touted as a very successful event. It served the participants well. I feel certain that it eventually served the patients well too, as they are the recipients of the care that is delivered. It was a one-day event that we worked hard to deliver, and we got satisfaction for a job well done. It was a team effort, and one that I drew on frequently during my career. It gave me self-confidence and self-satisfaction. I felt so good at the end of the conference when one of my co-workers looked at me, smiled, and said with certainty, "She has arrived." I will always remember this. An uplifting day with a satisfying ending.

This event was eliminated. This was seen to cut costs—just one example of the new "business approach" and cost-saving measures that trickled down to the nurses. Unfortunately, the cancellation also eliminated the opportunity for nurses to get together to organize and plan an energizing and educational event. It eliminated a day where nurses as professionals could be with other nurses to share ideas, discuss best practices, and make connections.

Pandemic 2020
Nancy's Story

It's been a very interesting time in recent months, working as a front-line nurse during the COVID-19 pandemic. I have had many people ask me about my "workday," as I currently work in an emergency department where this new virus is always on our minds, and it has changed many of our processes as we work with more rigorous infection-control practices. During the pandemic, with still no end in sight, I have had a lot of time to reflect on my work as a nurse and where we are today.

I've been working as a registered nurse now for twenty-seven years, having worked in several positions across the health system. Since the onset of the pandemic, nursing/front-line health care workers and the important work we do have been front and centre in this global fight against a virus that has truly become a significant part of all aspects of our daily lives. As a nurse, I have heard many inquiries and interest about nursing in the pandemic. Publicly, nurses have been thanked and recognized for the work we are doing and the risks we take every day in our work. My family, friends, acquaintances and the public are all applauding health care workers. This is wonderful and so important to keep our energy up. It has been gratifying and uplifting during this uncertain time for all.

FRONT LINE NURSING STORIES

When I graduated in the early 1990s, I was an enthusiastic twenty-three-year-old, grounded in nursing theory and all my newly acquired knowledge. It wasn't long into my first job that the reality of nursing really struck me. I worked in a hospital environment where there was truly a disconnect between the view I held of nursing, which was grounded in my formal education, and the realities of the work of a nurse. It wasn't long before I became quite disappointed in my work, realizing the disconnect between my likely idealistic views on nursing at that time and the actual reality of the work of a nurse. Since that time, I have done several different nursing roles. I have always been fortunate to find positions that have been interesting and flexible to allow me to raise a family and move to other roles easily. Today, I have returned to an acute care environment, which I left in the early days of my career, telling myself I would never go back.

Now I find myself working in a pandemic situation, where the past few months have been consumed with the potential for a surge of patients arriving at the hospital. The pandemic has brought to light the role and importance of the nurse and patient care in a time where safety is paramount, with a focus on infection-control practices. The public response has truly been unlike anything I have ever witnessed in my years of nursing. It has been a time where the public has truly shown their gratitude for the work we are doing.

It's now just past three months into the pandemic here at home. Day-to-day life is slowly opening, taking a staged approach. There is the "new normal" that seems to be the reality until a vaccine is available.

At work, "pandemic precautions" continue. Many of us are weary of our new work life reality and are yearning for our work to return to pre-COVID-19 times. The pandemic has truly put health care in the spotlight, highlighting the failures of our system over the years and revealing the disparities and vulnerabilities that have long been present in some of our systems of care.

Moving forward, there have been good moments and changes that have come out of the pandemic. There is a greater sense of "team "across all of us working in our department. I feel a renewed sense of energy about nursing and what we do and how important our work is. Politically, nurses need to keep pushing government to recognize the worth of our work. We must not be forgotten post-pandemic.

Although Nancy comments that the pandemic has put a "…. spotlight hightlighting the failures of our system…" nothing has really changed and some might argue that we may be regressing further in recognizing the value of the role of nursing. Two years into the pandemic the Ontario government passed bill 124 limiting the ability of nurses to negotiate salaries. Nancy's story also highlights the strong community support for nurses during this time. This theme is also present in the next two stories. Unfortunately strong community support for nursing during this time has not translated into more tangible formal benefits.

Nursing During COVID-19
Elaine's Story

Many different feelings and thoughts go through my head as I think about the pandemic and nursing in this past year.

Confusion, Safety Procedures, Comfort

Those masks and respirators, gowns and gloves, make me too hot. I can't breathe; I'm just too hot/sweaty; the moisture inside the respirators. I can't see, my glasses fogging up. My nose and ears are sore and I have pressure marks on my face from wearing masks.

There is no drinking/eating in any area other than the break room, which is not convenient or close. At the beginning of the pandemic, every vendor in the building was closed. Bathroom breaks were infrequent (not unusual: most nurses put it off in a normal day as we are just too busy), but in this case I wasn't drinking enough (so lack of hydration).

As time has moved along during this pandemic, we can be thankful we have enough personal protective equipment. Initially, we were reusing our masks during the shift and then putting them in bags labelled with our name—wiping off visors/goggles and reusing. We had limited supplies. We all long for the days when we won't have to wear masks. At least we hope those days will come again, or will they?

Fear and Disbelief

We didn't know what we were really dealing with at first, and the rules and procedures kept changing. I know a colleague or two who felt this was a hoax, a government conspiracy, even though they care for COVID patients. These people are the same people who have not gotten their vaccine yet. Some of my colleagues retired or quit due to worry for their own health, or due to a compromised parent or child/children or spouse at home. One of our pregnant nurses decided to stay home, due to concern for her unborn baby.

Uniforms were supplied so we didn't wear anything out of the hospital. Some of my co-workers would go home and strip their clothes off in the garage, then put them in a bag to launder while they showered. Some people had issues with rashes and dry irritated skin from shampooing and showering too frequently.

Helpless, No Control, Emotionally Drained

Our job has become more a function of priorities. Over the years, this has become a trend, but even more so now; often, our assignments have doubled. We have a sixteen-bed unit, but we had to surge to another unit to be able to ventilate more patients. We received ventilated patients from other areas in Ontario because they had no room, and the number of COVID patients was increasing quickly due to a variant outbreak. Our numbers have decreased some now—five weeks after another lockdown—and we have had some deaths, so we are back to our own unit. Staff are burned out. Some were doing overtime—that is, extra shifts and sometimes sixteen-hour days—along with doubled assignments to help manage the load.

Extra time is needed for donning and doffing, cleaning equipment, and seven people are needed to prone a patient. Extra time is needed for families. Since there is no visiting, they call for updates and want to Facetime. This is understandable: they want to see their loved one; they are worried and feel helpless and sometimes guilty. They are also isolated and lonely, wanting to talk to someone, even a stranger, such as a nurse. Some are struggling with COVID too. This is all very time-consuming and emotional.

Some of our COVID patients arrive already on life support; others can talk, be it one word at a time due to their shortness of breath and oxygen requirements. Some are struggling and are tired of working to breathe for days. They have heard the news and are now in an ICU, being told they need a tube and ventilator to help them with their breathing. They are frightened; you can see it in their eyes. You try to reassure them and you Facetime their family, so they can talk to them before they are sedated and put on a ventilator. They are aware this may be the last time they talk to their family. These people are my age or the age of my siblings, or my parents' age. Often their recovery is long, with multiple complications along the way: kidney failure, needing dialysis, a trach[eotomy] before getting off the vent, pressure sores from those hours of proning, and overall deconditioning from weeks or months on a vent. This is not to mention any underlying medical issues they had prior to COVID. Some do not survive, despite our efforts.

We need a break, at least until the next wave; the province relaxed the lockdown about two weeks ago.

Relief, Gratitude

We have had some COVID patients who became success stories. We lined the hall and clapped them out in the early days; their release was celebrated on the local TV news and in the paper. Now that the pandemic has been almost a year, patients go home without as much fanfare, but they are a success. They have made it home to be with their family. They are survivors.

Our community was so generous and willing to help. They donated money, masks, gloves—making hats and masks for us—and supplying food and coffee, which was so very much appreciated. There were thank-you cards and parades of support. We were called "heroes," which made me feel a little uncomfortable, since I do not consider myself a hero; I am just doing my job.

I have worked as an ICU nurse for thirty-seven years. These feelings I mention are not new, but the pandemic exaggerates them, and that affects the way I normally cope and deal with them. Unlike SARS, this pandemic is lengthy and has been especially difficult on everyone.

I Put Others First
Kelly S.'s Story

The COVID pandemic has most certainly affected me as a nurse in the most positive of ways. I work in the front line at a busy regional health centre in Ontario. COVID has forced me to acknowledge that every day I come to work, I decide to put others first. Not every day is going to be easy, but facing things head-on is the right thing to do. It has reminded me that even when I am scared, I can do meaningful work. I can decide to inspire, or I can succumb to my fear. I can decide to uplift instead of panic.

COVID has reminded me that we are all a small part of a much bigger picture. I have felt the love and respect from my community, a community that I serve with my entire heart each day. I have felt supported and respected by those I serve. They are scared and so am I. I acknowledge their fears, which helps me cast mine aside.

It has been and continues to be an enormous honour to serve others during this pandemic. I have always loved my work, and I am so very thankful that this pandemic has not taken that from me. I rely on my faith in God, my love for others, and the knowledge that I make a choice every day to decide to be thankful to get me through these difficult days.

Afterword

The stories in this book provide just a glimpse of the scope of nurses' experiences. The stories capture the tragedies and joys that confront nurses in the field. Through both tears and laughter, these stories show how nurses help turn tragedies into growth experiences for patients and their families. Some of the nurses share their own personal past and demonstrate how they have become stronger through their experiences. Death is not considered a happy occasion, but the stories about palliative care illustrate how peace can be derived as nurses support and coach patients and their families through the dying process.

Through the stories, we can discover the nurturing qualities of these healers. The nurses demonstrate their competence, connection, care, and compassion, their ability to listen, take risks, and just *be* with the patient. They show how, thanks to knowledge, education, perseverance, humanity, and caring, they have learned and developed these skills over time.

The stories tell the importance of good nurse–patient relationships to enhance the process of healing and transition. They identify obstacles to the development of this essential relationship, some of which are seen as systemic.

Although computers have added value in the health system, their introduction into the nursing assessment process can hamper relationship-building that is so important for healing. Some of the stories identify the horrific impact on both patient and nurse when there is inadequate funding to provide appropriate levels of care. Similarly, the nurse and, subsequently, the patients are negatively affected when they are not provided the proper supports after they experience traumatic events and as the workloads become overwhelming.

The stories make it abundantly clear that in the nursing profession, there are many specialty areas that a nurse can choose to work in. The stories I shared about my experiences indicate that my comfort level as a nurse in psychiatry is less than working in labour and delivery. This is not an indication of my abilities. It is an acknowledgment that some environments are more comfortable than other environments to work in. Brenda found it difficult to work with sick and dying children, as she found it too painful. Kerry told us that she very much enjoyed working with the "rough-and-tumble men of the woods." Some nurses are very effective and find it satisfying to support the patient and the family through the grieving and dying process.

Over the years, nurses have had to increase their education, skill sets, and knowledge bases to meet the expanding demands of the profession. The depth and breadth of knowledge have expanded to more effectively meet the needs of patients and their families. Nurses are in a pivotal position to know and understand patient needs and to identify gaps in services and care. They can and do advocate for patients, families, and communities within the health care system. The question is whether their voices are being adequately heard.

Throughout this book, there is a thread of dissatisfaction with the status of the nursing profession. Historically, we have been portrayed as unselfish caregivers without any expectations of meaningful compensation. The general public considers Florence Nightingale to be the Mother of Nursing. Sharon states unequivocally, "I am not Florence Nightingale," and she expects to be remunerated accordingly for the important work that she does as a nurse.

The time when nurses were considered the "handmaidens of doctors" no longer exists. Nursing has established itself as a profession, and it must be recognized as such. It is important for nurses to be valued partners, with a voice in the design and implementation of health care strategies to enhance health and healing for the patient. They must be recognized with adequate and appropriate compensation as well as provided the proper equipment to safely and effectively perform nursing roles. The culture and environments in which they work need to be supportive and empowering. It is not enough for nurses to be lauded as heroes during a pandemic and then forgotten. Nancy appreciates the accolades given to nurses during the ravages of COVID-19, but she fears that this recognition will disappear with the end of the pandemic.

In 2013, I signed up for a two-week mission to go to Kenya to help build the foundation of a school classroom. My husband and I went with a group of people from our local school board during my self-funded leave from work. Before going, I spoke with different people who had already done the trip or something similar. They said wonderful things about it all and described how it changed their lives. As a person who had been practising nursing for such a long time and in many different capacities, I was skeptical about how much it would change my life. I told myself that I had already seen so much pain, suffering, and illness because of my nursing career. I had my own personal experiences that often seemed so small compared to what many of my patients had to deal with in their lives. I thought that my life had been a bit different than most because I had been part of all these other lives. I had seen people acutely and chronically ill. I had seen families fall apart and hurt each other. I had seen them join in support. I had seen great leadership and leadership wanting. I had seen some poisonous working environments and some supportive ones.

I had worked with children and adults who needed protection from their families or friends. I had shared happiness with families and the birth of their children. I walked with patients and their families toward death. At times, I was inspired by the people in my care. I had felt amazed and at times helpless. I had seen the best and the worst in people and their behaviour toward each other. I have had many opportunities to make a difference. I have also had times when I felt I could have done better for people in my care by being more encouraging or more present.

Just when I thought I had seen it all, a new experience would present itself. I was open to the possibility that the Kenya experience might further expand my growth. I told myself that in going to Kenya, I would keep an open mind and heart. When asked why I wanted to go, I said, "I want to give back."

I had to stop and think. Did I really say that? At that point I recognized that my motivations to "give back" were clearly a statement of what nursing had given to me. I had been privileged to make this journey with my patients. It was a continual journey of self-reflection, self-discovery, and self-healing. Although there were lots of challenges along the way, meeting and overcoming them gave me strength and self-confidence. I was never bored and often amazed.

I slept and dreamt that life was joy.
I woke and saw that life was service.
I acted and behold, service was joy.
– Rabindranath Tagore

Printed in the USA
CPSIA information can be obtained
at www.ICGtesting.com
BVHW042241310723
668031BV00001B/4